Keys To An Amazing Life:

SECRETS OF THE CERVICAL SPINE

KENNETH K. HANSRAJ, M.D.

Keys To An Amazing Life: Secrets Of The Cervical Spine

©2012 by Dee Dee LLC

First Edition

Published by Dee Dee LLC

ISBN 978-0-9745374-1-2

Terms, Conditions and Disclaimers: Please read this agreement carefully before reading this book. By reading this disclaimer, you agree that you are competent and of age to enter into this Agreement and to be bound by the terms and conditions below. If you do not wish to be bound by these terms and conditions, you should not read or purchase this book. This information is presented as an educational service to the public. While the information is about health care issues and orthopaedic surgery, it is not medical advice. People seeking specific orthopaedic advice or assistance should contact an orthopaedic surgeon.

No Warranties: Although we believe the information in this book to be accurate and timely, because of the rapid advances in the field of orthopaedic surgery and our reliance on information provided by outside sources, we make no warranty or guarantee concerning the accuracy or reliability of the content of this book. When clinical matters are discussed in this book, the opinions presented are those of the discussants only. The material discussed in this book is not intended to present the only or necessarily the best orthopaedic method or procedure, but rather presents the approach or opinion of the discussant. This book and the information, software and other material available on or accessible from this book is provided on an "as is" and "as available" basis without warranties of any kind, expressed or implied, including but not limited to warranties of title, non-infringement or implied warranties of merchantability or fitness for a particular purpose. There is no warranty that the information will be uninterrupted or error free.

No Liability or Other Damages: Under no circumstances shall the author or publisher be liable for any direct, indirect, incidental, special, punitive or consequential damages that result in any way from your use of or inability to use this book, your reliance on or use of the information, services or merchandise provided on or through this book, or that result from mistakes, omissions interruptions, deletion of files, errors, defects, delays in operation, or transmission or any failure of performance. The author or publisher specifically disclaims any and all liability for injury and/or other damages that result from an individual using techniques discussed in this book, whether a physician or any other person asserts these claims.

Unauthorized Downloading or Distribution: Any unauthorized downloading and distribution of any copyrighted material from this book without the copyright owner's permission is strictly prohibited.

Indemnification: You agree to defend, indemnify and hold the author or publisher harmless from any and all liabilities, costs and expenses, including reasonable attorneys' fees, related to any violation of these terms and conditions by you.

Governing Laws and Venue: You agree to be bound by all applicable laws that may pertain to the book, including U.S. export and re-import laws and regulations. If any case or controversy arises regarding your use of the book, you agree that such case or controversy will be arbitrated or decided in the State of New York in the United States of America.

Changes in Terms and Conditions: The author and/or publisher reserves the right to change or modify these Terms and Conditions at any time, and you agree to give effect to such changes or modifications. By reading further, you acknowledge that you are aware of these.

Terms and Conditions: Please note that you understand these Terms and Conditions and that you agree to be bound by them. If you do not wish to be bound by these terms and conditions, you should not read and/or purchase this book.

DEDICATION

This book is dedicated to
my mom and dad
Augustus & Anjanie Hansraj

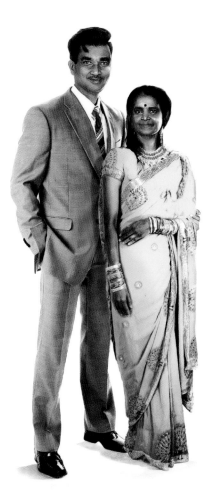

INTRODUCTION

WHEN I SIT DOWN TO CONSULT with a family member, dear friend or VIP from another country, a different set of words and concepts emerge from within me. I find it necessary to explain to them all of the factors that conspire to cause pain. "Did you know, based on MRI scans, that a significant percentage of people have spinal constrictions that would make a spinal surgeon feel the need to operate, even though those scans were taken of people that walk the planet everyday without pain," I ask. "Why do you have pain when they do not?"

It occurred to me that while people have various spinal defects, apparently certain unrelated conditions and human situations cause us to have or worsen this pain. Certain factors can inflame a previously tight nerve root and make it symptomatic. I observed that this is similar to turmoil in Nigeria causing elevated oil and gas prices in the United States of America. Therefore, I set out to perform, research and write a book to understand the factors that influence us to become susceptible to pain. I named this book "The Spinal Derivative." My friend Michael Yanko originally advised me to write a book that explains all the ways of "How To Never See Me In the Operating Room." My coach Dr. Todd Eller and his team at Business Breakthroughs International advised me to use a more "people friendly" name which became, *Keys to an Amazing Life: Secrets of The Cervical Spine.* This project took approximately four years to complete.

This research showed that 4 out of 5 humans do or will have a significant spinal problem in their lifetime. The incidence is fairly similar globally. Many countries do not have a way to assess how much they spend on spinal care, but the cost in the United States is approximately $100 billion per year. Studies show that education and awareness of spine health and its factors often leads to less pain and suffering.

This book introduces the non-medical reader to the anatomy of the spine in full-length illustrations followed by the specific parts of the spine. Gary Crumpler poured his heart into these renderings after he and I discussed how to bring the best concepts possible through beautiful and inspiring illustrations. Gary used 2.5D graphical techniques and shadowing to add depth and a gentle three-dimensional effect. I am grateful to Gary for his engaging, life-like illustrations.

I wrote the manuscript and my friend, Chris Miller, edited it for readability, grammar, and, especially, to make sure that all the concepts were explained.

Over time, I have developed a fascination and deep respect for the facet joints of the spine. Typical spinal problems are explained in great detail. Sixteen-year-old Robin Cornell read the manuscript and certified that it was fully legible to him. When the spine problems are explained, treatment and prevention options are shown.

Specific diagrams are presented to help the reader understand the individual nerves of the spine and their functions. The medical history and physical examination is fully explained and examples of findings on X-rays, MRI's, and CT-Myelograms are shown.

Human software, or the factors that run the inner self, is described. In this chapter, the intimate relationship of the spine and other organs of the body are explained. One can then understand the co-existence of spinal and general health. The power of a positive thought, random act of kindness, and the dangers of a negative thought were explained with a view through the body. The power of our thinking, imaginations, visualizations and actions are shown to be wired in our brain through modern concepts of neuroplasticity. The ability to change the size of our reptilian brain, the amygdala through meditation and its potential impact on spine health are explained. Full discussions of the factors that drive human happiness are also discussed.

Human hardware describes the mechanical factors in our hands. Positions, with good and bad postures, are shown and high-risk professionals, which include nurses, hairstylists, architects, laborers, welders and dentists are noted. Building designs influence human comfort with the potential for its inhabitants to experience less pain and suffering. Influences of water intake, hot and cold showers, wake-up time, sleep, nap, nerve and facet mobility are also discussed.

Social choices of cigarettes, alcohol, and prescribed or illicit drugs and their influence on spinal pain are examined.

Wholesome food options, aerobic activities, physical treatments, cervical stabilization, Osteopathic techniques, and Yoga techniques are shown.

Common pain management procedures and common anterior and posterior surgical procedures are illustrated and explained. Useful associated information is included in these chapters, such as how to prepare for surgery, medications that might cause bleeding, and the schedule for rehabilitation activities.

My mother and father encouraged me to be useful and helpful to humanity. Dad asked me a thousand times, "what is your purpose in life?" I am most grateful to my wife, physical medicine & rehabilitation specialist Marcia D. Griffin-Hansraj, D.O. for her help, thoughts and deep discussions on each chapter. My friends Gregory Chiaramonte, M.D., and Daniel Kelmanovich, M.D. helped me to create multiple four-hour windows to write this book. Numerous friends have encouraged me and engaged in the necessary and deep discussions. This is a partial list of the people to be thanked. Michael Yanko, Ninad Tipnis, Iman Mutlaq, Dermot Sweeny, Jacqueline Reeder, Christian Campilii, P.T., Todd Snyder, P.T., Robert Tomkins, D.O., Basil Abeysekara, M.D., Neera Jaspal, Jose Ramirez, Luc LeClerq, Patrick O'Leary, M.D., Nagendra Upadhyayula, M.D, David Gamburg, M.D., Srinivas Bonthu, M.D., Anthony Caramico, M.D., Gary Grossman, M.D. Thank you Alison Rayner for your remarkable book design. Photographers on this project were Jeff Karg, Michael Palumbo, Alan Shapiro, and myself.

Ken Hansraj, M.D.

Boden SD, McCowin PR, Davis DO, Dina TS, Mark AS, Wiesel S. *Abnormal magnetic-resonance scans of the cervical spine in asymptomatic subjects. A prospective investigation.* J Bone Joint Surg Am. 1990 Sep;72(8):1178-84.

TABLE OF CONTENTS

CHAPTER 1

*The
Global
Spinal Problem*

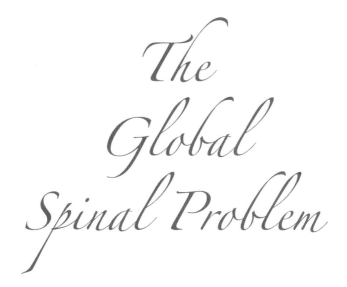

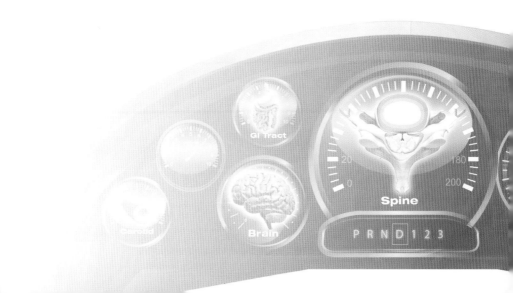

THE PROBLEM, EMERGING TRENDS, AND SOLUTIONS

NECK AND BACK PAIN are two of the most common reasons why people visit their doctor. According to the National Institute of Arthritis and Musculoskeletal and Skin Diseases, 8 out of 10 people suffer from some type of ailment to the spine, which results in either a constant, dull ache or a sudden, sharp pain.

In the United States, there is a wide variety of pain management options. A patient has the choice to first seek the expertise of a family doctor or an internist that, typically, apply gentle treatments, including medications or physical therapy, to ease the affected area. A vast majority of the time, these methods are highly successful.

Interaction with a chiropractor or a hands-on osteopathic physician as a source of primary care will often lead to treatments specific to their fields, which are quite effective. For example; spinal adjustments, soft tissue therapy, strength training, and nutritional recommendations are most often used by chiropractors, while mind-body interventions, biologically-based therapies, manipulative therapy, and energy therapies are common among osteopathic physicians.

IN THE UNITED STATES OF AMERICA:

$560 to 635 billion dollars: The total cost of pain to society in 2010.

$309 billion dollars: The cost of heart disease in 2010.

$243 billion dollars: The cost due to cancer in 2010.

$188 billion dollars: The cost of diabetes in 2010.

Institute of Medicine of the National Academies, July 2011

The physicians of the Physical Medicine and Rehabilitation field are well suited to treat pain and suffering due to back and neck problems, especially from a function restoration point of view. A neurologist, on the other hand, is a nerve specialist that is quite adept in diagnosing and rendering treatment options in spinal care. A referral is made to a surgeon if pain still persists after less invasive options have been exhausted.

A patient's choice and a general physician's referral of an Orthopedic or Neuro Spinal surgeon is usually based upon the reputation and experience of the surgeon. In terms of training and ability, both choices are equally qualified to address spinal problems.

My recommendation for surgery candidates is to search for a board certified surgeon that only specializes in spine care. Listen with the heart. If a good rapport with the surgeon is established, then move ahead. If not, then keep shopping.

The more specialized the spine specialist, unfortunately, the more difficult it is to acquire an appointment. After charting history, performing a physical examination, and reviewing the magnetic resonance imaging (MRI) tests, there could be as little as only 10 minutes remaining in the appointment to discuss the spinal problem. This leaves no chance to compile a comprehensive assessment of all the factors that could help remedy the condition.

This book was written from my heart, with the patient in mind, to be a source of understanding of every factor that I have found to be imperative in the alleviation of suffering due to spinal pain. While I certainly enjoy being able to surgically bring relief to those with back and neck problems, I am happy to teach people the importance of deep breathing and meditation. Both exercises lead to better sleep and significant pain relief.

Often times, patients can learn what triggers their back pain and refrain from the activity or body position or posture, resulting in never requiring surgery. In contrast, far too many people are ignorant to the destructive effects cigarette smoking has on the intervertebral disc.

I am content to render care for a patient that learns the importance and strategies of weight loss, followed by spine stabilization and proper strengthening of the muscles of the back and neck.

The bottom line: In most cities in the United States, people have an overwhelming number of specialists from which to choose, while in rural settings they can run scarce. Globally, there are approximately 300 million people with access to great healthcare, while billions do not have physician options. Many countries have only one spine specialist or, possibly, none at all.

Based upon my 15 years and more than 20,000 consults rendered as a spinal surgeon, with over 2,000 spinal operations performed, I decided to write this book. My goal is to help the interested person understand the factors that contribute to the health and well-being of the spine.

While this book is specifically about the neck, low back pain studies are more common and are used to discuss the various drivers.

COSTS OF SPINE PAIN

More United States health care dollars are spent treating spinal problems than most other medical conditions. Specific data is difficult to obtain, but estimated medical costs associated with back and neck pain increased by 65% between 1997 and 2005, to approximately $86 billion. Current estimates of the annual economic impact of back and neck pain in the United States is in excess of $100 billion.

While international costs related to back pain are even more difficult to find and estimate, one economic study reported that the indirect costs of back pain within the whole labor force in 1991 in the Netherlands were estimated between $2 billion and $4.5 billion.

GLOBAL PREVALENCE OF SPINE PAIN

Within every 3 month period in the United States, approximately 25% of adults report having low back pain (LBP). Chronic pain present in the adult population ranges from 15% to 40%. LBP is defined as chronic after 3 months. Distress arising from various structures of the spine accounts for a majority of the chronic pain disorders. The average person has a 60% to 80% chance of developing significant back and neck pain within their lifetime. Richard A. Deyo, M.D., M.P.H., professor and Kaiser-Permanente Endowed Professor of Evidence-based Medicine in the Department of Family Medicine at Oregon Health and Science University, conducted studies among racial groups. His findings revealed that American Indians and Alaskan Natives have the highest prevalence of LBP, while Asian Americans have the lowest occurrence.

According to the National Health Survey of 2002-2003, more than 50% of the French population in the 30 to 64 year-old age group experienced back pain at least one time, with 17% reported experiencing back pain for more than 30 days in the previous 12 months.

The predominance of low back pain, as assessed by the National Health Survey, was similar to that found in countries other than France. In the Afyon region of Turkey, lifetime LBP prevalence was 51% and chronic LBP prevalence was 13%. Overall, 63% of women and 34% of men experienced LBP at least one time in their lives.

With 12-month prevalence rates of more than 70%, back pain is currently a major health problem for German adults, and one that entails major economic consequences.

Australia developed the National Health Priority Area initiative to promote cooperation between government and non-government organizations to monitor, report on, and develop strategies to improve health outcomes for its people. Upwards of 80% of Australians encounter back pain at some point in their lives. As a result, 10% of those affected will experience significant disability.

There is a general assumption that the predominance of LBP is lower in Africa, comparatively, than it is in developed countries. A review of 27 eligible epidemiological studies out of Africa concluded that the prevalence of spinal pain is rising and similar to the rest of the world.

SEX DIFFERENCE

Epidemiological surveys have readily reported that women are more frequently, and more severely, affected by LBP than men. Women are also more likely to encounter recurrent or chronic low back pain.

THE CONTRIBUTION OF SMOKING
TO NECK AND BACK PAIN

Smoking cigarettes is universally recognized as a major contributor to back pain. As evidenced by recent data, 1.5 pack years, or approximately 550 packs, of cigarette smoke in 18-year-old girls was the threshold for LBP consultation. One pack year equals 365 packs of cigarettes and is calculated by multiplying 1 pack (20 cigarettes) per day for 1 year, or 2 packs (40 cigarettes) per day for half a year, and so on.

There is significant psychiatric literature indicating smoking's link to suicidal ideation (thoughts of killing oneself, with or without a plan and/or an intent). Studies concluded that the number of cigarettes smoked per day correlated with a smoker's chief complaint of suicidal ideations. The data suggested that suicidal ideations increased if the patient smoked heavily and had continuing problems with alcohol. Newer literature is beginning to describe the incremental effects of smoking in better detail.

THE ROLE OF EXERCISE

Physical activity is important and is often suggested for the prevention and management of low back pain. However, both inactivity and excessive activity increase the risk of developing back pain. An increasing number of triathletes have presented with various spinal disorders attributed to overuse. Gymnasts, alpine skiers and runners are also examples of athletes that run the risk of back and neck problems and its repercussions.

Typists are required to maintain a sitting position for extended periods of time. In this group, one study suggested that the subjects were able to identify that at least one hour of exercise per week significantly reduced LBP prevalence. A separate study showed that one hour of strenuous physical activity, weekly, proved to be beneficial in protecting seniors from back pain.

ASSOCIATED MEDICAL PROBLEMS

Arterial plaque formation can obstruct branching arteries of the abdominal aorta, including four, paired lumbar arteries and the middle sacral artery that feeds the lumbar spine. Diminished blood flow to these areas could result in various back problems. Carotid artery inner lining (intima-media) thickness was found to be associated with continuous, radiating low back pain among women and men, and with a positive unilateral clinical sign of sciatica in men only.

Studies performed on a relatively young population concluded that abdominal obesity might increase the risk of LBP in women. More specifically, a high body mass index, waist circumference, hip circumference, waist-to-hip ratio, serum leptin level (hormone involved in fat metabolism), and C-reactive protein level (a marker for inflammation) were related to an increased prevalence of low back pain in women.

Stress biomarkers in patients with chronic pain have known to be associated with stress-related disorders as well as health and recovery. Individuals with a high level of regenerative/anabolic activity have less pain than those that do not. Decreased regenerative/anabolic activity is associated with increased pain. The big message is that muscle building, fitness, and regeneration protect from pain.

A variety of inflammatory mediators of pain are being identified and others have already been implicated in the degeneration of the intervertebral disc, including nitric oxide (NO), interleukins, matrix metalloproteinases (MMP), prostaglandin E2 (PGE2), tumor necrosis factor alpha (TNF-alpha), and a group of cytokines. MMPs, PGEs, and a variety of cytokines have already been proven to play a role in the degradation of articular cartilage. NO is a novel mediator that has recently drawn much attention for its role in disc abnormalities. Elevated

NO production derived from nitric oxide synthase (NOS) activity has been manifested in cerebrospinal spinal fluid in patients with degenerative lumbar disease. These specific mediators could lead to innovations of future treatments.

GENETICS

Prior research has demonstrated the existence of a familial predisposition to internal disc degeneration with a, generally, high heritability. Segregation analysis, a method to determine whether a trait is genetic by testing whether the transmission pattern in human families is consistent with Mendelian expectations (i.e., dominant, recessive, or codominant), has demonstrated that the mode of inheritance is complex with multiple factors and genes involved in intergenerational transmission.

EMOTIONAL AND MENTAL FACTORS

Study evaluators are consistently impressed how emotional and mental factors significantly contribute to the presence and severity of back and neck pain. Depression magnifies pain, which can cause anxiety, irritability, and agitation. Depression and anxiety, along with chronic pain, is associated with experiencing more severe pain, greater disability, and a poorer health-related quality of life. Besides workplace ergonomics, employee satisfaction and happiness are important factors to consider with patients that suffer from back and neck pain syndromes.

ROLE OF EDUCATION
OF THE HUMAN BEING

Recent investigations were recently conducted between education level and low back pain in the adult population, especially concerning the role of physical working constraints and personal factors such as weight, tobacco use, and height. LBP was found to be strongly associated with education level. Those less educated about back pain factors were found to experience more LBP.

Culture and ethnic background, along with factors such as intelligence and diabetes-related obesity, plays a significant role in back and neck pain suffering. Investigations have made it clear that certain groups of people will be more likely to experience pain from spinal problems as a result of cultural norms. For example, those which emphasize less exercise and embrace a poor diet.

This book helps
to level the playing field.

BIBLIOGRAPHY

Altinel L, Köse KC, Ergan V, Işik C, Aksoy Y, Ozdemir A, Toprak D, Doğan N. *[The prevalence of low back pain and risk factors among adult population in Afyron region, Turkey].* Acta Orthop Traumatol Turc. 2008 Nov-Dec;42 (5): 328-33. Turkish.

Andrusaitis SF, Oliveira RP, Barros Filho TE. *Study of the prevalence and risk factors for low back pain in truck drivers in the state of São Paulo, Brazil.* Clinics (Sao Paulo). 2006 Dec;61(6):503-10.

Bair MJ, Wu J, Damush TM, Sutherland JM, Kroenke K. *Association of depression and anxiety alone and in combination with chronic musculoskeletal pain in primary care patients.* Psychosom Med. 2008 Oct;70(8):890-7. Epub 2008 Sep 16.a

Balousek S, Plane MB, Fleming M. *Prevalence of interpersonal abuse in primary care patients prescribed opioids for chronic pain.* J Gen InternMed. 2007 Sep;22(9):1268-73. Epub 2007 Jul 20.

Bertram H, Nerlich A, Omlor G, Geiger F, Zimmerman G, Fellenberg J. *Expression of TRAIL and the death receptors DR4 and DR5 correlates with progression of degeneration in human intervertebral disks.* Mod Pathol. 2009 Jul;22(7):895-905. Epub 2009 Mar 20.

Betrisey D. *Labor, social exclusion and chronic muscular illness: the case of mid-impoverished sectors in a peripheral neighborhood in Madrid, Spain.* Med Anthropol. 2009 Jan-Mar; 28 (1): 65-80

Bracci M, Croce N, Baldassari M, Amati M, Monaco F, Santarelli L. *[Low back pain in VDT operators: importance of sports activities].* G Ital Med Lav Ergon. 2007 Jul-Sep;29 (3 Suppl): 563-4. Italian.

Briggs, AM, Buchbinder R. *Back pain: a National Health Area in Australia?* Med J Aust. 2009 May 4;190(9) :499-502.

Buchbinder R, Staples M, Jolley D. *Doctors with a special interest in back pain have poorer knowledge about how to treat back pain.* Spine (Phila Pa 1976). 2009 May 15;34(11)1218-26;discussion 1227.

Cakmak A (1); Yücel B (2); Özyalcin SN (3); Bayraktar B (4); Ural HI (1) ; Duruöz MT (5); Genc A (2); Spine 2004, vol. 29, no14, pp. 1567-1572 [6 page(s) (article)] (22 ref.)

Carey TS, Freburger JK, Holmes GM, Castel L, Darter J, Agans R, Kalsbeek W, Jackman A. *A long way to go: practice patterns and evidence in chronic low back pain care.* Spine (Phila Pa 1976). 2009 Apr 1;34(7) : 718-24.

Chenot JF, Becker A, Leonhardt C, Keller S, Donner-Banzhoff N, Hildebrandt J, Basler HD, Baum E, Kochen MM, Pfingsten M. *Sex differences in presentation, course, and management of low back pain in primary care.* Clin J Pain. 2008 Spe;24 (7):578-84.

Dagenais S, Caro J, Haldeman S. *A systematic review of low back pain cost of illness studies in the United States and internationally.* Spine J. 2008 Jan-Feb; 8(1): 8-20. Review.

Deyo RA, Mirza SK, Martin Bl. *Back pain prevalence and visits rates: estimates from U.S. national surveys, 2002.* Spine (Phila Pa 1976). 2006 Nov 1;3 (23) : 2724-7

Eubanks JD, Lee MJ, Cassinelli E, Ahn NU. *Prevalence of lumbar facet arthrosis and its relationship to age, sex, and race: an anatomic study of cadaveric specimens.* Spine (Phila Pa 1976). 2007 Sep 1;32(19):2058-62.

Fathallah FA, Miller BJ, Miles JA. *Low back disorders in agriculture and the role of stooped work; scope, potential interventions, and research needs.* J Agric Saf Health. 2008 Apr;14(2): 221-45. Review.

Fenga C, Tringali M, Fenga D, Di Nola C, Drago M. *Column and upper limb musculoskeletal disorders in drivers helpers.* G Ital med Lav Ergon. 2007 Jul-Sep; 29 (3 Suppl):585-6. Italian.

Fishbain DA, Lewis JE, Gao J, Cole B, Steele Rosomoff R. *Are chronic low back pain patients who smoke at a greater risk for suicide ideation?* Pain Med. 2009 Mar;10(2) :340-6. Epub 2009 Feb 25.

Forcier L, Lapointe C, Lortie M, Buckle P, Kuorinka I, Lemaire J, Beaugrand S. *Supermarket workers: their work and their health, particularly their self-reported musculoskeletal problems and compensable injuries.* Work. 2008;30 (4) :493-510.

Franklin GM, Stover BD, Turner JA, Fulton-Kehoe D, Wickizer TM; Disability Risk Identification Study Cohort. *Early opioid prescription and subsequent disability among workers with back injuries: the Disability Risk Identification Study Cohort.* Spine (Phila Pa 1976). 2008 Jan 15;33 (2):199-204.

Freburger JK, Holmes GM, Agans RP, Jackman AM, Darter JD, Wallace AS, Castel LD, Kalsbeek WD, Carey TS. *The rising prevalence of chronic low back pain.* Arch Intern Med. 2009 Feb 9; 169(3):251-8.

Friese CR, Abel GA, Magazu LS, Neville BA, Richardson LC, Earle CC. *Diagnostic delay and complications for older adults with multiple myeloma.* Leuk Lymphoma. 2009 Mar;50(3):392-400.

Fullen BM, Baxter GD, O'Donovan BG, Doody C, Daly L, Hurley DA. *Doctors' attitudes and beliefs regarding acute low back pain management: A systematic review.* Pain. 2008 Jun;136(3):388-96. Epub 2008 Apr 18. Review.

Gagnier JJ, van Tulder MW, Berman B, Bombardier C. *Herbal medicine for low back pain: a Cochrane review.* Spine (Phila Pa 1976). 2007 Jan 1;32 (1):82-92 Review. Erratum in: Spine. 2007 Aug 1;32(17):1931

Gepstein R, Arinzon Z, Folman Y, Shabat S, Adunsky A. *Lumbar spine surgery in Israeli Arabs and Jews: a comparative study with emphasis on pain perception.* Isr Med Assoc J. 2007 Jun;9(6):443-7.

Gnudi S, Sitta E, Gnudi F, Pignotti E. *Relationship of a lifelong physical workload with physical function and low back pain in retried woman.* Aging Clin Exp Res. 2009 Feb;21(1) :55-61.

Gourmelena J, Chastanga J-F, Ozgulera A, Lanoëa J-L, Ravaudb J-F and Leclerca A. *Annales de Réadaptation et de Médecine Physique,* Volume 50, Issue 8, November 2007, Pages 640-644

Guh DP, Zhang W, Bansback N, Amarsi Z, Birmingham CL, Anis AH. *The incidence of co-morbidities related to obesity and overweigh; a systematic review and meta-analysis.* BMC Public Health. 2009 Mar 25; 9:88. Review.

Harden RN, Remble TA, Houle TT, Long JF, Markov MS, Gallizzi MA. *Prospective, randomized, single-blind, sham treatment-controlled study of the safety and efficacy of an electromagnetic field device for the treatment of chronic low back pain: a pilot study.* Pain Pract. 2007 Sep;7(3): 245-55.

Hartvigsen J, Christensen K. *Active lifestyle protects against incident low back pain in seniors: a population-based 2-year prospective study of 1387 Danish twins aged 70-100 years.* Spine (Phila Pa 1976). 2007 Jan 1;32(1):76-81.

Heneweer H, Vanhees L, Picavet HS. *Physical activity and low back pain: a U-shaped relation?* Pain. 2009 May;143 (1-2) :21-5. Epub 2009 Feb 12.

Hides JA, Stanton WR, McMahon S, Sims K, Richardson CA. *Effect of stabilization training on multifidus muscle cross-sectional area among young elite cricketers with low back pain.* J Orthop Sports Phys Ter. 2008 Mar;38(3):101-8. Epub 2007 Dec 7.

Holguin N, Muir J, Rubin C, Judex S. *Short applications of very low-magnitude vibrations attenuate expansion of the intervertebral disc during extended bed rest.* Spine J. 2009 Jun;9(6): 470-7. Epub 2009 Apr 8.

Jang R, Karwowski W, Quesada PM, Rodrick D, Sherehiy B, Cronin SN, Layer JK. *Biomechanical evaluation of nursing tasks in a hospital setting.* Ergonomics. 2007. Nov;50(11):1835-55.

Janwantanakul P, Pensri P, Jiamjarasrangsi W, Sinsongsook T. *Associations between prevalence of self-reported musculoskeletal symptoms of the spine and biopsychosocial factors among office workers.* J Occup Health. 2009;51(2): 114-22. Epub 2009 Feb 3.

Janwantanakul P, Pensri P, Jiamjarasrangsri V, Sinsongsook T. *Prevalence of self-reported musculo-skeletal symptoms among office workers.* Occup Med (Lond). 2008 Sep;58(6):436-8. Epub 2008 Jun 10.

Jensen TS, Karppinen J, Sorensen JS, Niinimäki J, Leboeuf-Yde C. *Vertebral endplate signal changes (Modic change): a systematic literature review of prevalence and association with non-specific low back pain.* Eur Spine J. 2008 Nov;17 (11): 1407-22. Epub 2008 Sep 12. Review.

Kalichman L, Hunter DJ. *The genetics of intervertebral disc degeneration. Familial predisposition and heritability estimation.* Joint Bone Spine. 2008 Jul;75(4): 383-7. Epub 20008 Apr 29. Review.

Kalko Y, Kafa U, Başaran M, Köşker T, Ozçalişkan O, Yücel E, Aydin U, Yaşar T. *Surgical experiences in acute spontaneous dissection of the infrarenal abdominal aorta.* Anadolu Kardiyol Derg. 2008 Aug;8(4) : 286-90.

Kalso E, Simpson KH, Slappendel R, Dejonckheere J, Richarz U. *Predicting long-term response to strong opioids in patients with low back pain: finders from a randomized, controlled trial of transdermal fentanyl and morphine.*

Karahan A, Kav S, Abbasoglu A, Dogan N. *Low back pain: prevalence and associated risk factors among hospital staff.* J Adv Nurs. 2009 Mar;65(3): 516-24.

Kauppila LI. *Atherosclerosis and disc degeneration/low-back pain—a systematic review.* Eur J Vasc Endovasc Surg. 2009 Jun;37(6):661-70. Epub 2009 Mar 27. Review.

Khoueir P, Black MH, Crookes PF, Kaufman HS, Katkhouda N, Wang MY. *Prospective assessment of axial back pain symptoms before and after bariatric weight reduction surgery.* Spine J. 2009 Jun;9(6):454-63. Epub 2009 Apr 8.

Knaepen K, Cumps E, Zinzen E, Meeusen R. *Low-back problems in recreational self-contained underwater breathing apparatus divers; prevalence and specific risk factors.* Ergonomics. 2009 Apr; 52(4):74+61-73.

Lee H, Wilbur J, Kim MJ, Miller AM. *Psychosocial risk factors for work-related musculoskeletal disorders of the lower-back among long-haul international female flight attendants.* J Adv Nurs. 2008 Mar;61(5): 492-502.

Lorusso A, Bruno S, Caputo F, L'Abbate N. *[Risk factors for musculoskeletal complaints among microscope workers]*. G Ital Med Lav Ergon. 2007 Oct-Dec; 29(4): 932-7. Italian.

Lorusso A, Bruno S, L'Abbate N. *A review of low back pain and musculoskeletal disorders among Italian nursing personnel*. Ind Health. 2007 Oct;45(5): 637-44. Review.

Louw QA, Morris LD, Grimmer-Somers K. *The prevalence of low back pain in Africa: a systematic review*. BMC Musculoskelet Disord. 2007 Nov 1;8:105. Review.

Manchikanti L, Singh V, Datta S, Cohen SP, Hirsch JA. *Comprehensive review of epidemiology, scope, and impact of spinal pain*. American Society of Interventional Pain Physicians. Pain Physician. 2009 Jul-Aug;12(4):E35-70.

Manchikanti L, Singh V, Datta S, Cohen SP, Hirsch JA. *Comprehensive review of epidemiology, scope, and impact of spinal pain*. American Society of Interventional Pain Physicians. Pain Physician. 2009 Jul-Aug;12(4):E35-70.

Marx P, Püschmann H, Haferkamp G, Busche T, Neu J. *Manipulative treatment of the cervical spine and stroke]*. Fortschr Neurol Psychiatr. 2009 Feb;77(2):83-90. Epub 2009 Feb 16. German.

Mikkonen P, Leino-Arjas P, Remes J, Zitting P, Taimela S, Karppinen J. *Is smoking a risk factor for low back pain in adolescents? A prospective cohort study*. Spine (Phila Pa 1976). 2008 Mar 1;33(5): 527-32.

Miller D, Richardson D, Eisa M, Bajwa RJ, Jabbari B. *Botulinum Neurotoxin-A for Treatment of Refractory Neck Pain: A Randomized, Double-Blind Study*. Pain Med. 2009 Jul 6.

Miyamoto M, Konno S, Gembun Y, Liu X, Minami K, Ito H. *Epidemiological study of low back pain and occupation risk factors among taxi drivers*. Ind Health. 2008 Apr; 46(2): 112-7.

Mok Lc, Lee IF. *Anxiety, depression and pain intensity in patients with low back pain who are admitted to acute care hospitals*. J Clin Nurs. 2008 Jun;17(11);1471-80. Epub 2009 Feb 19.

Oleske DM, Lavender SA, Andersson GB, Kwasny MM. *Are back supports plus education more effective than education alone in promoting recovery from low back pain?: Results from a randomized clinical trial*. Spine (Phila Pa 1976). 2007 Sep 1;32(19):2050-7.

Palmer KT, Harris CE, Griffin MJ, Bennett J, Reading I, Sampson M, Coggon D. *Case-control study of low-back pain referred for magnetic resonance imaging, with special focus on whole-body vibration*. Scand J Work Environ Health. 2008 Oct;34(5):364-73. Epub 2008 Oct 14. Erratum in: Scand J Work Environ Health. 2009. Jan;35 (1) 80. Harris, E Claire [corrected to Harris, E Claire].

Petersen T, Larsen K, Jacobsen S. *One-year follow-up comparison of the effectiveness of McKenzie treatment an strengthening training for patients with chronic low back pain: outcome and prognostic factors*. Spine (Phila Pa 1976). 2007 Dec 15;32(26):2948-56.

Plouvier S, Renahy E, Chastang JF, Bonenfant S, Leclerc A. *Biomechanical strains and low back disorders: quantifying the effects of the number of years of exposure on various types of pain*. Occup Environ Med. 2008 Apr;65 (4):268-74. Epub 2007 Oct 10.

Podichetty VK. *The aging spine: the role of inflammatory mediators in intervertebral disc degeneration*. CellMol Biol (Noisy-le-grand). 2007 May 30;53(5):4-18. Review.

Prady Sl, Thomas K, Esmonde L, Crouch S, MacPherson H. *The natural history of back pain after a randomized controlled trial of acupuncture vs usual care—long term outcomes.* Acupunct Med. 2007 Dec;25(4):121-9.

Quiroz-Moreno R, Lezama-Suárez G, Gómez-Jiménez C. *[Disc alterations of lumbar spine on magnetic resonance images in asymptomatic workers].* Rev Med Inst mex Seguro Soc. 2008 Mar-Apr; 46(2): 185-90. Spanish.

Roelofs PD, Deyo RA, Koes BW, Scholten RJ, van Tudler MW. *Nonsteroidal anti-inflammatory drugs for low back pain: an updated Cochrane review.* Spine (Phila Pa 1976). 2008 Jul 15;33(16):1766-74. Review.

Rossignol M, Abouelfath A, Lassalle R, Merlière Y, Droz C, Bégaud B, Depont F, Moride Y, Blin P, Moore N, Fourrier-Règlat A. *The CADEUS study: burden of nonsteroidal anti-inflammatory drug (NSAID) utilization for musculoskeletal disorders in blue collar workers.* Br J Clin Pharmacol. 2009 Jan;67 (1) : 118-24.

Rubin DI. *Epidemiology and risk factors for spine pain.* Neurol Clin. 2007May;25(2):353-71. Review

Schell E, Theorell Tr, Hasson D, Arnetz B, Saraste H. *Stress biomarkers' associations to pain in the neck, shoulder, and back in healthy media workers: 12-month prospective follow-up.* Eur Spine J. 2008 Mar;17(3):393-405. Epub 2007 Dec 13.

Schmidt CO, Raspe H, Pfingsten M, Hasenbring M, Basler HD, EichW, Kohlmann T. *Back pain in the German adult population: prevalence, severity, and sociodemographic correlates in a multiregional survey.* Spine (Phila Pa 1976). 2007 Aug 15;32(18):2005-11.

Schnedier S, Randoll D, Buchner M. *Why do women have back pain more than men? A representative prevalence study in the federal republic of Germany.* Clin J Pain. 2006 Oct;22(8):738-47.

Shipp EM, Cooper SP, del Junco DJ, Delclos Gl, Burau KD, Tortolero S, Whitworth RE. *Chronic back pain and associated work and non-work variables among farmworkers from Starr County, Texas.* J Agromedicine. 2009;14(1): 22-32.

Shiri R, Solovieva S, Husgafvel-Pursiainen K, Taimela S, Saarikoski La, Huupponen R, Viikari J, Raitakari OT, Viikari-Juntura E. *The association between obesity and the prevalence of low back pain in young adults: the Cardiovascular Risk in Young Finns Study.* Am J Epidemiol. 2008 May 1;167(9):1110-9. Epub 2008 Mar 11.

Shiri R, Viikari-Juntura E, Leino-Arjas P, Vehmas T, Varonen H, Moilanen L, Karppinen J, Heliövaara M. *The association between carotid intima-media thickness and sciatica.* Semin Arthritis Rheum. 2007 Dec;37(3):174-81. Epub 2007 May 15.

Shiue HS, Lu CW, Chen CJ, Shih TS, Wu SC, Yang CY, Yang YH, Wu TN. *Musculoskeletal disorder among 52,261 Chinese restaurant cooks cohort: result from the National Health Insurance Data.* J Occup Health. 2008 Mar;50(2): 163-8.

Skoffer B. *Low back pain in 16-16 year old children in relation to school furniture and carrying of the school bag.* Spine (Phila Pa 1976). 2007 Nov 15;32(24):E713-7.

Smith L, Louw Q, Crous L, Grimmer-Somers K. *Prevalence of neck pain and headaches: impact of computer use and other associative factors.* Cephalalgia. 2009 Feb;29(2):250-7.

Spyropoulos P, Papathanasiou G, Georgoudis G, Chronopoulos E, Koutis H, Koumoutsou F. *Prevalence of low back pain in greek public office workers.* Pain Physician. 2007 Sep;10(5): 651-9.

Sun J, He Z, Wang S. *[Prevalence and risk factors of occupational low back pain in ICU nurses].* Zhonghua Lao Dong Wei Sheng Zhi Ye Bing Za Zhi. 2007 Aug;25(8): 453-5. Chinese.

Sung PS, Lammers AR, Danial P. *Different parts of erector spinae muscle fatigability in subjects with and without low back pain.* Spine J. 2009 Feb;9(2):115-20. Epub 2008 Feb 14.

Tiemessen IJ, Hulshof CT, Frings-Dresen MH. *Low back pain in drivers exposed to whole body vibration: analysis of a dose-response pattern.* Occup Environ Med. 2008 Oct;(10):667-75. Epub 2008 Jan 23.

Urquhart DM, Bell R, Cicuttini FM, Cui J, Forbes A, Davis SR. *Low back pain and disability in community-based women: prevalence and associated factors.* Menopause. 2009 Jan-Feb;16(1):24-9.

Urquhart DM, Hoving JL, Assendelft WW, Roland M, van Tudler MW. *Antidepressants for non-specific low back pain.* Cochrane Database Syst Rev. 2008 Jan 23;(1):CD001703. Review.

Van Nieuwenhuyse A, Crombez G, Burdorf A, Verbeke G, Masschelein R, Moens G, Mairiaux P; BelCoBack Study Group. *Physical characteristics of the back are not predictive of low back pain in healthy workers: a prospective study.* BMC Musculoskelet Disord. 2009 Jan5; 10:2.

Verbunt JA, Sieben J, Vlaeyen JW, Portegijs P, Andre Knottnerus J. *A new episode of low back pain: who relies on bed rest?* Eur J Pain. 2008 May; 12(4):508-16. Epub 2007 Sep 17.

Villavicencio AT, Burneikiene S, Hernández TD, Thramann J. *Back and neck pain in triathletes.* Neurosurg Focus. 2006 Oct 15;21(4):E7.

Voorhies RM, Jiang X, Thomas N. *Predicting outcome in the surgical treatment of lumbar radiculopathy using the Pain Drawing Score, McGill Short Form Pain Questionnaire, and risk factors including psychosocial issues and axial joint pain.* Spine J. 2007 Sep-Oct; 7(5):516-24. Epub 2007 Jan 2.

Wasan AD, Jamison RN, Pham L, Tipirneni N, Nedeljkovic SS, Katz JN. *Psychopathology predicts the outcome of medical branch blocks with corticosteroid for chronic axial low back or cervical pain: a prospective cohort study.* BMC Musculoskelet Disord. 2009 Feb 16;10:22.

Waters T, Genaidy A, Barriera Viruet H, Makola M. *The impact of operating heavy equipment vehicles on lower back disorders.* Ergonomics. 2008 May;51(5): 602-36. Review.

Weidenhammer W, Streng A, Linde K, Hoppe A, Melchart D. *Acupuncture for chronic pain within the research program of 10 German Health Insurance Funds—basic results from an observational study.* Complement Ther Med. 2007 Dc;15(4):238-46. Epub 2006 Oct 30.

Wenig CM, Schmidt CO, Kohlmann T, Schweikert B. *Costs of back pain in Germany.* Eur J Pain. 2009 Mar;13(3):280-6. Epub 2008 Jun 3.

Wilkey A, Gregory M, Byfield D, McCarthy PW. *A comparison between chiropractic management and pain clinic management for chronic low-back pain in a national health service outpatient clinic.* J Altern Complement Med. 2008 Jun;14(5):465-73.

Witt CM, Pach D, Brinkhaus B,Wruck K, Tag B, Mank S,Willich SN. *Safety of acupuncture: results of a prospective observational study with 229,230 patients and introduction of a medical information and consent form.* Forsch Komplementmed. 2009 Apr; 16(2):91-7. Epub 2009 Apr 9.

Yoshioka K, Toribatake Y, Kawahara N, Tomita K. *Acute aortic dissection or ruptured aortic aneurysm associated with back pain and paraplegia.* Orthopedics. 2008 Jul;31(7):651.

CHAPTER 2

*Anatomy
of the Spine*

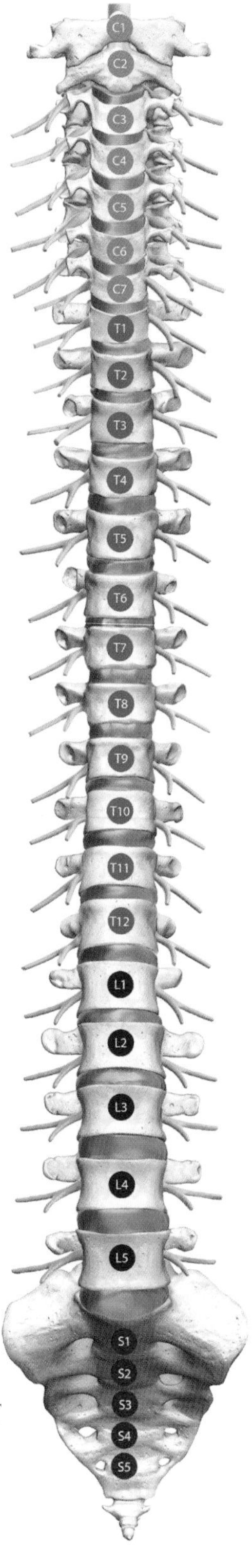

FRONT
VIEW

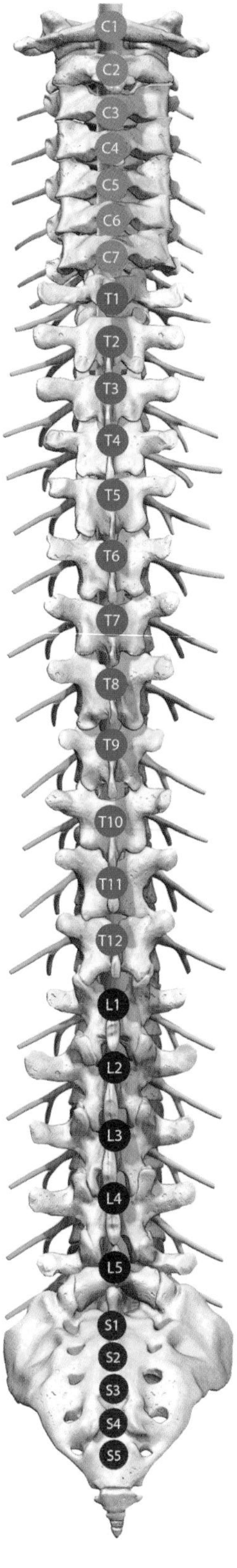

BACK
VIEW

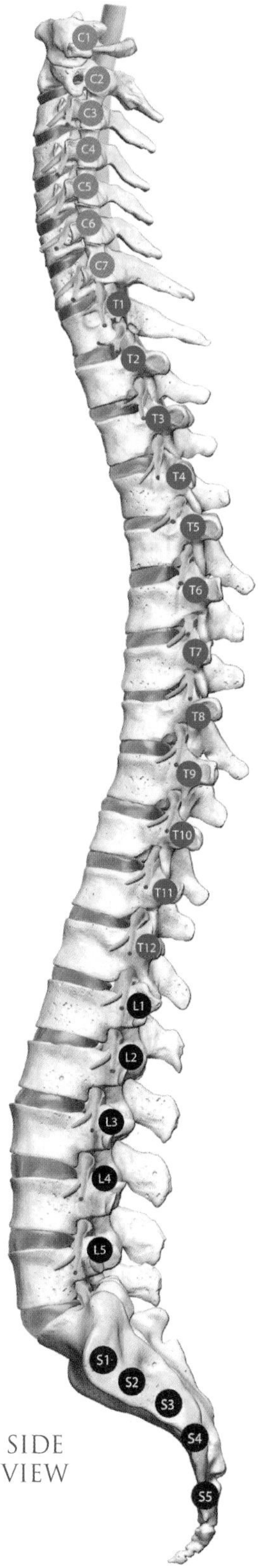

The spinal column is comprised of:

7 Cervical Vertebrae called the neck
12 Thoracic Vertebrae called the mid-back
5 Lumbar Vertebrae called the back
1 Sacrum called the tail-bone
1 Coccyx called the distal tail-bone

SIDE
VIEW

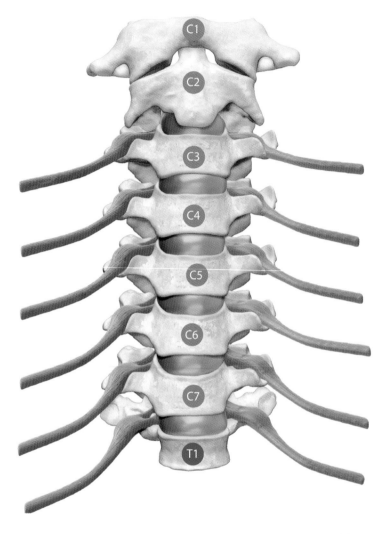

THIS IS A VIEW OF THE FACE OF THE FRONT OF THE CERVICAL SPINE.

The C1 and C2 carry a different look and function than the C3, C4, C5, C6, and C7.

The C1 and C2 control most of the side by side rotation of the cervical spine (e.g., the ability to rotate your neck to the sharp right and sharp left).

The C2, C3, C4, C5, C6, and C7 are shown with discs, vertebral bodies, and exiting nerves.

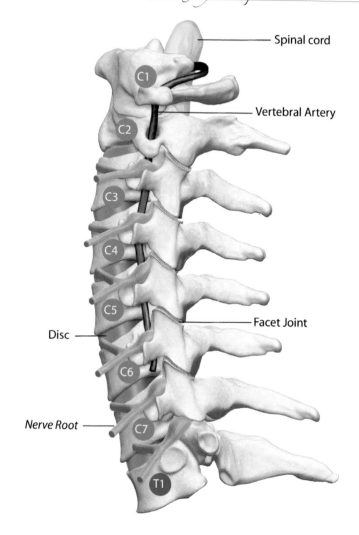

Spinal cord

Vertebral Artery

Facet Joint

Disc

Nerve Root

C1

C2

C3

C4

C5

C6

C7

T1

THIS IS A SIDE VIEW OF THE CERVICAL SPINE.

The C1 and C2 carry a different look and function than the C3, C4, C5, C6, and C7.

The all-important vertebral artery is shown traveling through the neck. This artery supplies oxygen to the brainstem and vital parts of the brain.

The C1 and C2 control most of the side by side rotation of the cervical spine.

The C2, C3, C4, C5, C6, and C7 are shown with discs, vertebral bodies and exiting nerves.

The facet joints are noted in the back of the spine.

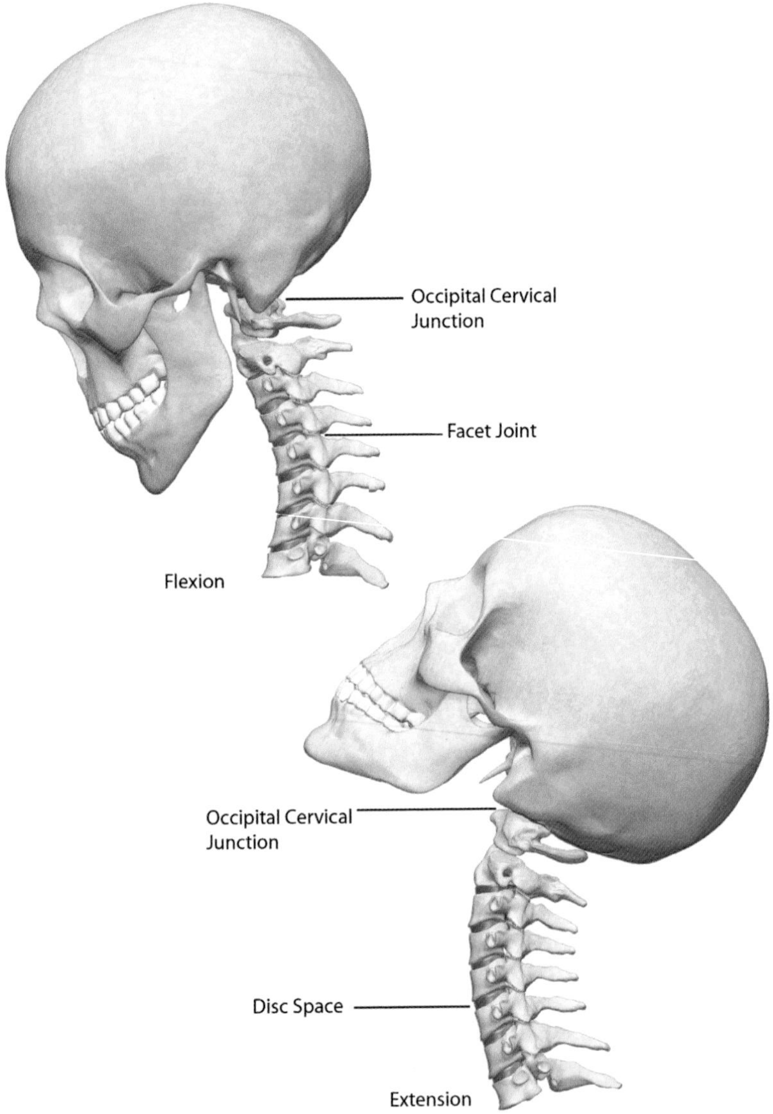

Occipital Cervical Junction

Facet Joint

Flexion

Occipital Cervical Junction

Disc Space

Extension

Occiput to C1 (the occipital-cervical junction) determines 50% of the upward and downward motion of the neck, called flexion and extension. Note the amount of natural motion through the disc spaces and facet joints. This rendering started with flexion-extension X-rays of a 30 year old female patient. The images were captured from the X-rays showing motion of flexion and extension and then illustrated. Therefore, this is a real-time study.

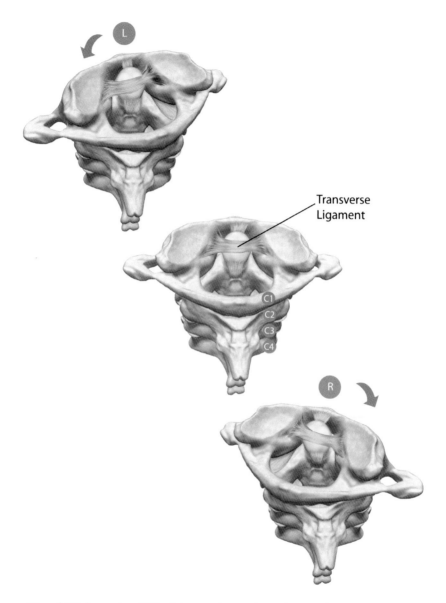

Transverse Ligament

C1
C2
C3
C4

L

R

C1 and C2 determines 50% of the rotation as shown here in these images. The remainder of the 50% of the motion is shared through the C2-3, C3-4, C4-5, C5-6, and C6-7. These lower levels levels (C2-3, C3-4, C4-5, C5-6, and C6-7) account for approximately 10% of the side by side motion, per level.

POSTERIOR ELEMENTS

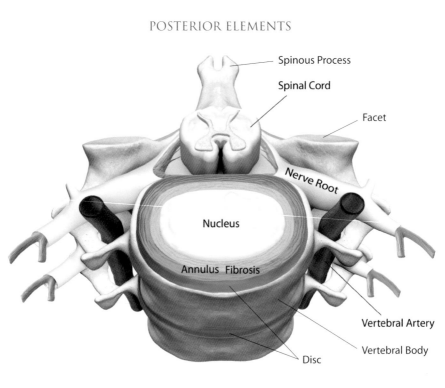

Spinous Process

Spinal Cord

Facet

Nerve Root

Nucleus

Annulus Fibrosis

Vertebral Artery

Vertebral Body

Disc

ANTERIOR ELEMENTS

The disc sits between two vertebral bodies. The anterior elements of the spine consists of the vertebral bodies and the disc space in between. The disc consists of an outer circumferential layer called the annulus fibrosis. Think of the annulus as the Great Wall of China surrounding and protecting the nucleus pulposus. The annulus has 2 layers of collagen which protects the nucleus with two axes of strength. The nucleus pulposus is a lobular soft tissue shock absorber.

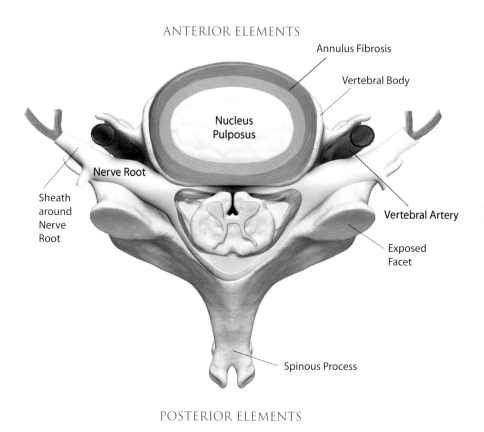

ANTERIOR ELEMENTS

Annulus Fibrosis

Vertebral Body

Nucleus Pulposus

Nerve Root

Sheath around Nerve Root

Vertebral Artery

Exposed Facet

Spinous Process

POSTERIOR ELEMENTS

The posterior elements of the spine consists of the spinal canal with the spinal cord and nerve roots, as well as the facet joints, lamina and spinous processes.

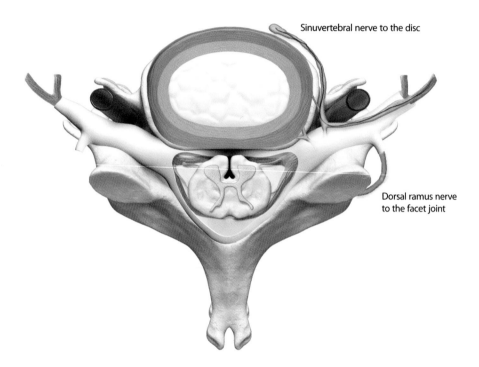

Sinuvertebral nerve to the disc

Dorsal ramus nerve to the facet joint

Nerves in the disc often accompany blood vessels and here demonstrated being branches of the sinuvertebral nerve to the disc, itself, and the dorsal ramus to the facet joint.

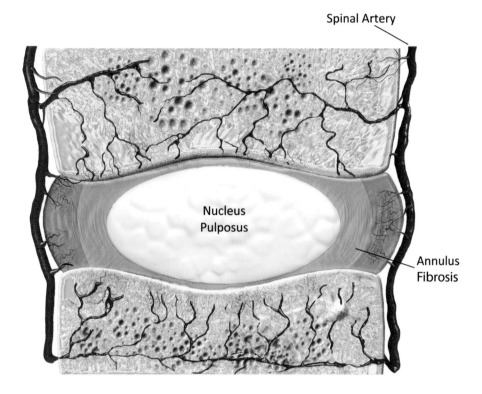

The blood supply to the disc space is tenuous at best. This diagram shows the blood vessels present in the longitudinal ligaments adjacent to the disc. When one studies the limited blood supply to the disc, it becomes easy to understand that further compromise will lead to rapid breakdown of the disc spaces. Only the outer third of the annulus fibrosis received blood supply.

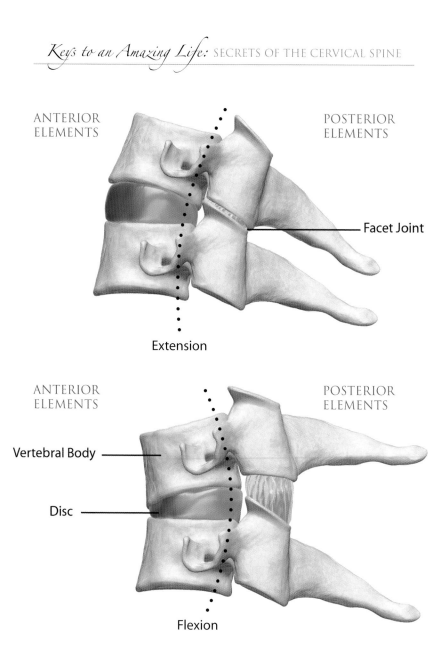

ANTERIOR ELEMENTS

POSTERIOR ELEMENTS

Facet Joint

Extension

ANTERIOR ELEMENTS

POSTERIOR ELEMENTS

Vertebral Body

Disc

Flexion

The facet joints are the keystone of the spine. They provide motion and are truly no different than the hip and knee joints. Facet joints have capsules and joint fluids. Strategies for servicing these joints are also helpful in the function of the neck.

Athletes, especially, need to employ ways to warm up, service, and provide range of motion to their facet joints. Special attention to the facet joint will help prevent pain and suffering as well as enhance life and career.

CHAPTER 3

Typical Spinal Problems

CERVICAL STRAIN/SPRAIN
CERVICAL HERNIATED DISCS
CERVICAL DEGENERATIVE DISC DISEASE
CERVICAL STENOSIS
CERVICAL INFECTION
CERVICAL TUMOR

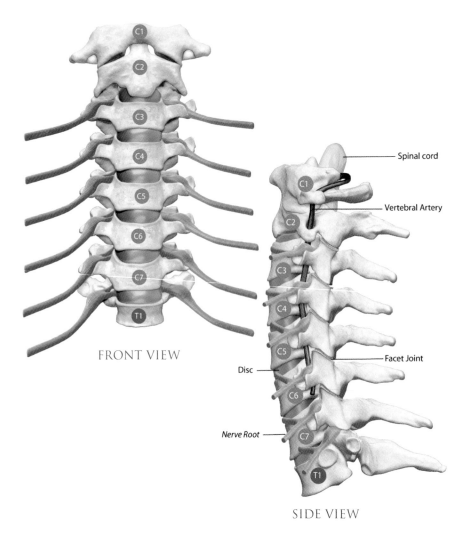

FRONT VIEW

SIDE VIEW

THE NORMAL HUMAN INTERVERTEBRAL DISC

The normal disc is a combination of strong connective tissues that hold one vertebra to the next and serves as a cushion. This human shock absorber consists of a tough outer layer called the annulus fibrosis and a gel-like center called the nucleus pulposus.

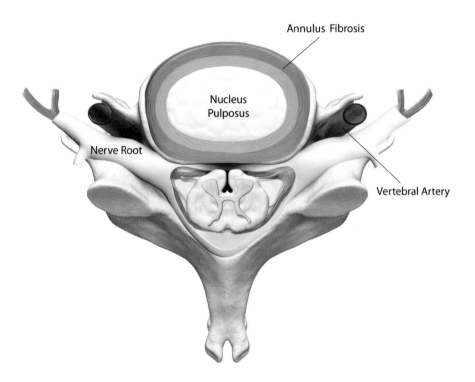

The normal cervical human intervertebral disc consists of an annulus fibrosis that has an external layer and an internal layer which surround and protect the shock absorber, the nucleus pulposus. This figure shows the spinal cord with bilateral nerves exiting through the nerve channels called neuroforamen. The essential vertebral artery is shown in red.

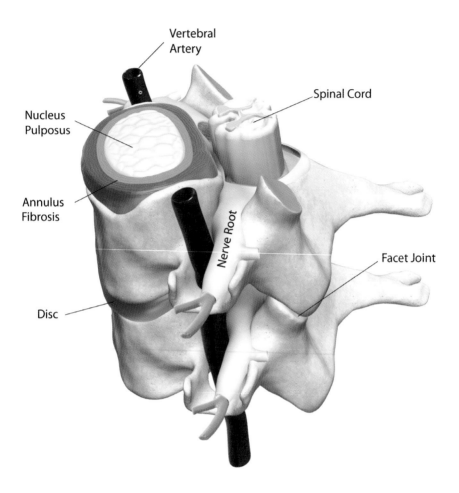

This figure illustrates the normal cervical human intervertebral disc from the side view. It shows the spinal cord with nerves exiting through the neuroforamen. The important vertebral artery is shown in red. The vertebral artery branches from the subclavian artery, runs through the neck and supplies significant portions of the posterior brain.

CERVICAL STRAIN
& SPRAIN

CERVICAL STRAIN AND SPRAIN refers to injuries concerning the ligaments, arteries, veins, muscles, and nerves of the neck. Technically, a sprain is an injury involving the stretching or tearing of ligaments, while strains are injuries that involve the stretching or tearing of muscle and tendon structure. I inform my patients that their vital and precious structures are most likely bruised and stretched, yet full recovery is expected.

Traditional treatments include early motion, traction, physical therapy, massage, modalities (i.e. ice, heat, tens/sequential stimulation, and ultrasound), acupuncture, osteopathic manipulations, chiropractic care, pain management (epidural versus selective nerve root blocks), activity avoidance, and activity and job modifications. Heat in the form of long, hot showers, saunas, and heat packs can help relieve pain. Application of cold packs and gels could also offer some relief. Medications in the classes of aspirin, non steroidal anti-inflammatories, muscle relaxants, oral steroids, antidepressants, and narcotics might be recommended. External stabilization in the form of a brace could be helpful in the short term.

When the patient is less symptomatic, specific treatments such as cervical stabilization will often assist with the resumption of function and endurance. Yoga and Pilates may be used to strengthen and stabilize muscles, while Medx treatment (an aggressive program consisting of three phases, each comprising a maximum of six dynamic strength exercise sessions) might help strengthen neck muscles.

HERNIATED
NUCLEUS PULPOSUS
AKA SLIPPED DISC OR HERNIATED DISC

THE NORMAL DISC is a combination of strong connective tissue that connects one vertebra to the next. This human shock absorber consists of a tough outer layer called the annulus fibrosis. A herniated disc exists when the gel-like center called the nucleus pulposus exits through a hole caused by damage to the annulus fibrosis.

Classically, the patient complains of neck pain and a sharp, lancing pain progressing distally from the neck, shoulder blade and shoulder into the arm in a specific zone. Radiculopathy refers to the irritation of a nerve root, causing symptoms (pain, numbness, weakness, plus/minus reflex changes) in the zone of the nerve root.

Numbness, tingling or weakness of the leg is called sciatica. Similar symptoms may be experienced in the arms or around the trunk.

Loss of bowel or bladder control is an emergency.
Seek immediate medical attention!

Traditional treatments include early motion, traction, physical therapy, massage, modalities, acupuncture, osteopathic manipulation, chiropractic care, pain management, activity avoidance, and activity with job modifications. Heat in the form of long, hot showers, sauna, and heat packs can help reduce pain. Application of cold packs and gels could also offer some relief. Medications in the classes of aspirin, non steroidal anti-inflammatories, muscle relaxants, oral steroids, antidepressants, and narcotics could also be recommended. External stabilization in the form of a brace might prove to be beneficial in the short term.

When the patient is less symptomatic, specific treatments such as cervical stabilization will often assist with the resumption of function and endurance. Yoga and Pilates may be used to strengthen core muscles, while Medx treatment might help to strengthen neck muscles.

Cervical injections such as epidural steroid, facet blocks, or radiofrequency ablation may be recommended.

Cervical spine (neck) surgical treatments include anterior cervical discectomy and fusion (ACDF) and posterior foraminotomy or decompression, fusion and instrumentation.

Prevention: While wear, tear, and breakdown of the discs is natural and unavoidable, certain factors will accelerate the process. Repetitive bending, lifting, twisting, reaching, vibration exposure, poor posture, poor body mechanics, weak abdominal and extensor muscles, smoking, and obesity can increase the rate of disc breakdown. An appreciation of the cervical facet joint's anatomy could, specifically, help in the long-term preservation of neck function. Understanding the function, motion and limitations of the facet joint can serve as a tool to help slow the process of wear and tear in the neck.

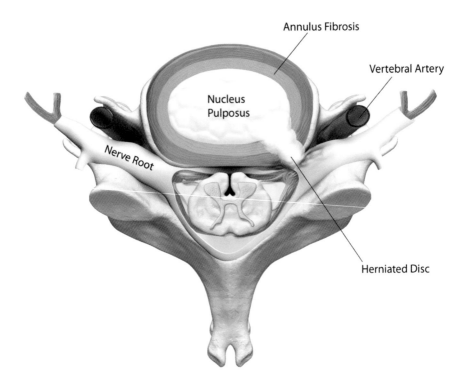

Annulus Fibrosis

Vertebral Artery

Nucleus
Pulposus

Nerve Root

Herniated Disc

VIEW OF A HERNIATED DISC

A herniated disc occurs when the nucleus pulposus exits through the annulus fibrosis. Notice that the nerve is mechanically compressed and inflamed.

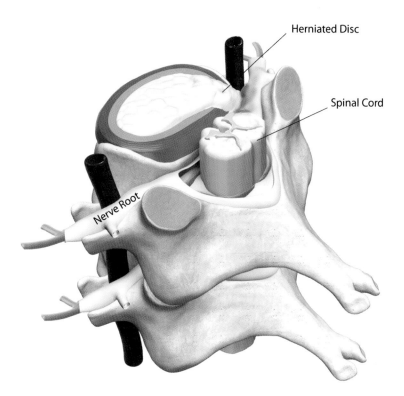

Herniated Disc

Spinal Cord

Nerve Root

THIS FIGURE DISPLAYS A LARGE HERNIATED DISC FROM A SIDE VIEW

Notice the nucleus pulposus exits through the annulus fibrosis.

DEGENERATIVE DISC DISEASE
AKA BLACK DISC DISEASE

DEGENERATIVE DISC DISEASE describes the wear and tear of the disc. Degenerative disc disease is a misnomer for the reason that it sounds as though it's a progressive and threatening condition. This process occurs naturally with age. However, it is not strictly degenerative and is not actually a disease. Degenerative disc disease can also be accelerated by a motor vehicle accident or labor and other repetitive activities, known as traumatic degeneration. The basic problem begins with a tear in the fibers that make up the annulus fibrosis. It is recognized that annular tears cause pain by excreting inflammatory chemicals that are caustic to nerve roots and neural elements. The break down and the collapse of the facet joints cause mechanical pain.

Classically, a patient with this condition complains of neck pain through the scapula (shoulder blade), which is exacerbated by sitting or standing. The pain is commonly reported as being deep, dull, and aching, or a boring pain, progressing distally from the neck into the arm in a nonspecific zone. This is as opposed to radiculopathy, which is an irritation of the nerve root. Pain, numbness, weakness, and +/− reflex changes of the arm might be present.

Loss of bowel or bladder control is an emergency.
Seek immediate medical attention!

Traditional treatments include early motion, traction, physical therapy, massage, modalities, acupuncture, osteopathic manipulation, chiropractic care, pain management, activity avoidance, and activity with job modifications. Heat in the form of long, hot showers, sauna, and heat packs can help relieve pain. Application of cold packs and gels could also offer some relief. Medications in the classes of aspirin, non steroidal anti-inflammatories, muscle relaxants, oral steroids, antidepressants, and narcotics might be recommended. Wearing a brace for external stabilization could be helpful in the short term.

When the patient is less symptomatic, specific treatments such as cervical stabilization will often assist with the resumption of function and endurance. Yoga and Pilates may be used to strengthen core muscles, while Medx treatment might help to strengthen neck muscles.

Cervical injections such as epidural steroid, facet blocks, or radiofrequency ablation may be recommended.

Cervical spine surgical treatments include ACDF and posterior foraminotomy or decompression, fusion and instrumentation.

Prevention: While wear, tear, and break down of the discs is natural and unavoidable, certain factors will accelerate the process. Repetitive bending, lifting, twisting, reaching, vibration exposure, poor posture, poor body mechanics, weak abdominal and extensor muscles, smoking, and obesity can increase the rate of disc break down. An appreciation of the cervical facet joint's anatomy could, specifically, help in the long-term preservation of neck function. Understanding the function, motion, and limitations of the facet joint can serve as a tool to help slow the process of wear and tear in the neck.

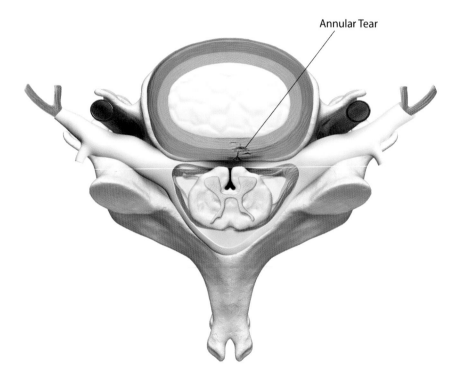

Early degenerative disc disease represents a process of tears in the annulus shown here on the axial view.

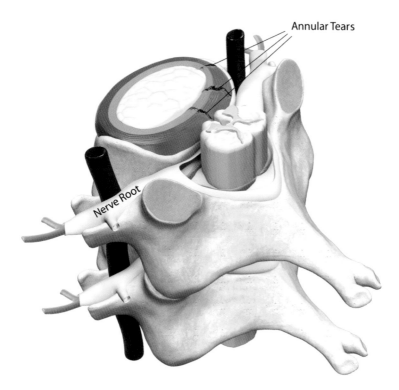

Annular Tears

Nerve Root

SIDE VIEW OF THE SPINE WITH
THREE ANNULAR TEARS NOTED

With further wear and tear, multiple annular tears may be expressed.

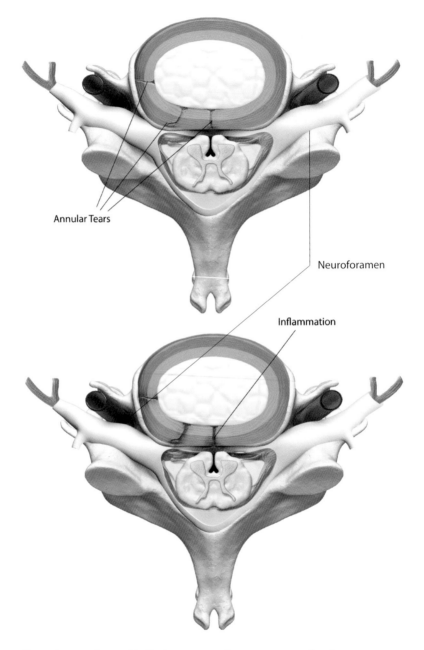

From time to time, with further wear and tear, more annular damage occurs. These annular tears may spill inflammatory mediators with chemical irritation of the nerve roots and the spinal cord.

CERVICAL SPINAL STENOSIS

S PINAL STENOSIS OCCURS when there is arthritic buildup that blocks the spinal channels. This causes a narrowing of the spinal canal and/or nerve canal. The central canal, which carries the spinal cord, and both neuroforamen comprise the three main channels. Arthritic spurs build up on the facet joints in the posterior portion of the spine due to activity, time, wear, and tear. These arthritic spurs begin to encroach on the nerve channels and pinch the nerve roots. This usually occurs in the neck (cervical), mid-back (thoracic), and the lower back (lumbar).

Cervical stenosis patients might present with spinal cord (upper motor neuron symptoms) and/or with nerve root symptoms. Stiffness or weakness of the hands, lower greater than upper limb weakness, a broad-based shuffling gait, lower extremity numbness, incoordination of the limbs, radiating lightning-like sensations down the back due to neck flexion and, although rare, bowel and bladder changes could occur.

The bottom two levels of the cervical spine (C5-6 and C6-7) are the most commonly involved, which is confirmed and diagnosed with an MRI or CT scan/myelogram.

Traditional treatments include early motion, traction, physical therapy, massage, modalities, acupuncture, osteopathic manipulation, chiropractic care, pain management, activity avoidance, and activity with job modifications. Heat in the form of long, hot showers, sauna, and heat packs can help relieve pain. Application of cold packs and gels could also offer some relief. Medications in the classes of aspirin, non steroidal anti-inflammatories, muscle relaxants, oral steroids, antidepressants, and narcotics could also be recommended. External stabilization in the form of a brace might prove to be beneficial in the short term.

When the patient is less symptomatic, specific treatments such as cervical stabilization will often assist with the resumption of function and endurance. Yoga and Pilates may be used to strengthen core muscles, while Medx treatment might help to strengthen neck muscles.

Cervical injections such as epidural steroid, facet blocks, or radiofrequency ablation may be recommended.

Cervical spine surgical treatments include anterior cervical discectomy and fusion (ACDF) and posterior foraminotomy or decompression, fusion and instrumentation.

Prevention: While wear, tear, and break down of the discs is natural and unavoidable, certain factors accelerate the process. Repetitive bending, lifting, twisting, reaching, vibration exposure, poor posture, poor body mechanics, weak abdominal and lumbar extensor muscles, smoking, and obesity can increase the rate of disc breakdown. An appreciation of the cervical facet joint's anatomy could, specifically, help in the long-term preservation of neck function. Understanding the function, motion, and limitations of the facet joint can serve as a tool to help slow the process of wear and tear in the neck.

SIDE VIEW OF THE CERVICAL SPINE

Side view of the cervical spine shows the convergence of degenerative disc disease and stenosis. As the disc degenerates and breaks down, the disc space collapses, the nerve channel called the neuroforamen becomes smaller and stenotic with impingement.

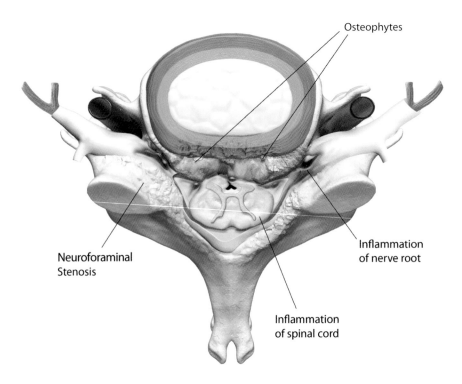

Osteophytes

Inflammation
of nerve root

Neuroforaminal
Stenosis

Inflammation
of spinal cord

THIS FIGURE SHOWS CENTRAL (AND NEUROFORAMINAL) STENOSIS OF THE SPINAL CORD.

Wear, tear, and age could cause the spinal canal and cord to become restricted in space. Constricting the spinal cord at such a high level might lead to upper motion neuron signs such as stiffness or weakness of the hands, lower greater than upper extremity weakness, a broad-based shuffling gait, incoordination of either or both lower or upper limbs, lower extremity numbness, radiating lightning-like sensations down the back due to neck flexion, and although rare, bowel and bladder changes.

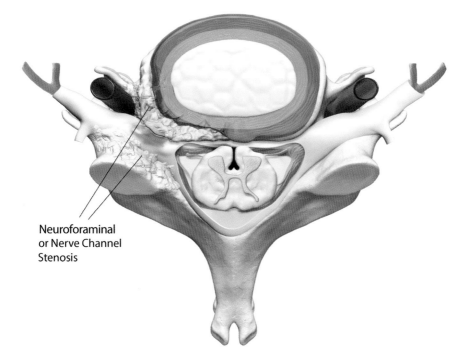

Neuroforaminal
or Nerve Channel
Stenosis

THIS FIGURE SHOWS
NEUROFORAMINAL STENOSIS OF THE NERVE ROOT.

Lateral or neuroforaminal stenosis is caused by constriction of a nerve as it exits the nerve channel. Nerve root symptoms, known as radiculopathy, describes the pain, weakness, and +/− numbness that could manifest in the distribution of a nerve root.

For example, a right-sided C6 radiculopathy might cause weakness in the right bicep and brachioradialis (forearm) muscle, numbness in the C6 distribution (thumb and index finger), and diminished reflexes in the brachioradialis tendon.

SPONDYLOLISTHESIS

(*SPONDYLOS* » VERTEBRA, *OLISTHESIS* » TO SLIP)

SPONDYLOLISTHESIS is a condition in which one vertebral body is slipped over another. This is predominantly a problem of the lumbar spine, although slippage of the vertebral body can occur throughout the spine.

Traditional treatments include early motion, traction, physical therapy, massage, modalities, acupuncture, osteopathic manipulation, chiropractic care, pain management, activity avoidance, and activity and job modifications. Heat in the form of long, hot showers, sauna, and heat packs can help relieve pain. Application of cold packs and gels could also offer some relief. Medications in the classes of aspirin, non steroidal anti-inflammatories, muscle relaxants, oral steroids, antidepressants, and narcotics might be recommended. External stabilization in the form of a brace might prove to be beneficial in the short term.

When the patient is less symptomatic, specific methods such as cervical stabilization will often assist with the resumption of function and endurance. Yoga and Pilates may be used to strengthen core muscles, while Medx treatment might help to strengthen neck muscles.

Cervical spine surgical treatments include ACDF and posterior foraminotomy or decompression, fusion and instrumentation.

Prevention: While wear, tear, and break down of the discs is natural and unavoidable, certain factors accelerate the process. Repetitive bending, lifting, twisting, reaching, vibration exposure, poor posture, poor body mechanics, weak abdominal and extensor muscles, smoking, and obesity can

GRADE	% SLIP
1	1-24%
2	25-49%
3	50-74%
4	75-99%
5	100%

increase the rate of disc breakdown. An appreciation of the cervical facet joint's anatomy could, specifically, help in the long-term prevention of neck function. Understanding the function, motion, and limitations of the facet joint can serve as a tool to help slow the process of wear and tear in the neck.

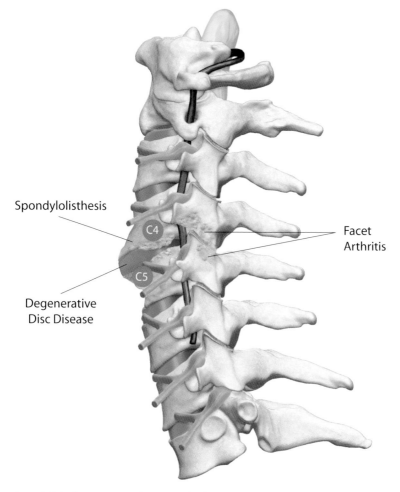

Spondylolisthesis is a condition in which one vertebral body is slipped over the other. Ligaments loosen, facets deteriorate, discs collapse, and forward slippage of the spine can occur due to aging, wear, tear, and trauma.

Multiple spinal problems tend to occur in late cases all at once. Along with spondylolisthesis, there is associated degenerative disc disease and facet arthritis.

CERVICAL INFECTION

CERVICAL SPINE INFECTIONS typically affects the patient by causing pain, tiredness, fevers, and chills. X-rays and MRI scans could show a collection of fluid as shown here. Lab work such as a CBC (complete blood count), an ESR (erythrocyte sedimentation rate), and a CRP (c-reactive protein – protein blood levels which rise in response to inflammation) gauges the level of infection. Treatment includes washing out the area in surgery and removing any of the obvious sources of infection. Cultures are taken during surgery. Depending on the organism, an infectious diseases specialist recommends a specific course of antibiotic therapy.

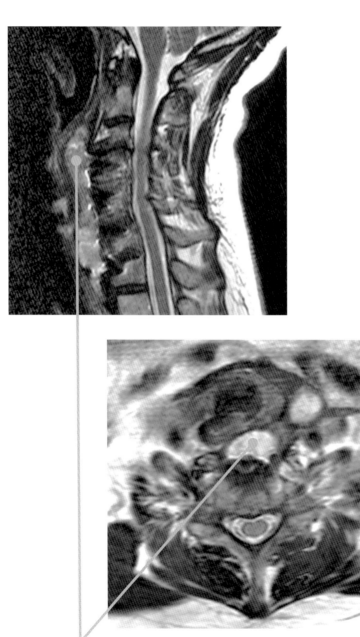

A collection of fluid is shown after an anterior cervical reconstruction.
Further blood testing with a CBC, ESR and a c-reactive protein (CRP)
showed an infection.

CERVICAL TUMOR

THIS IS A CASE REPORT of a patient with Paget's disease with sarcomatous transformation of the cervical spine vertebra. This is the second ever reported case in the world literature.

The patient, an 82-year-old man, complained of a feeling of pins and needles in his hands and arms. Worsening neck pain and stiffness, difficulty with balance, and pain on right side of the head and shoulders for 3-4 months was noted. He had night pain, and he was unable to walk due to poor balance, as well as an inability to stand well and drive.

Physical examination showed his head flexed forward due to an excessive curvature of the thoracic spine, known as a kyphotic posture or kyphosis. He presented with decreased reflexes in both upper extremities, which was much worse on the right at 1 out of 4, compared to the left side at 1+/4. He demonstrated weakness in both upper extremities, rated about 3 out of 5 and being bilaterally worse in C7 and C8.

Laboratory evaluation showed elevated alkaline phosphatase levels.

Radiographs of the cervical spine taken by the patient's chiropractor demonstrated Pagetoid involvement of C2 including the dens and of the lamina of C2. There was no apparent sarcomatous degeneration at that point. After six months, the lamina was extremely thick with evidence of sarcomatous tumor involvement. An MRI scan of the cervical spine revealed that there was a 6 x 3.5cm. mass destroying the posterior elements of C2 and C3. CT of the cervical spine demonstrated a bone forming lesion on the lamina of C2. Whole body bone scan showed that the Paget's disease was involved in the left humerus bone of the arm and the pelvis.

The tumor was resected and the spine was stabilized with an occipital cervical construct and bone fusion, using surgical strategies shown in the posterior cervical spine surgery chapter.

Although primary tumors of the cervical spine are rare, they must be thought of in cases with persistent pain. Patients with cervical spine tumors report having chronic pain, especially through the night. Patients could experience weight loss and fevers might be present. Tumors that originate from the spinal cord and nerves are called primary spinal tumors. Sometimes, with other cancers, a tumor will spread to the spine. This is called a metastatic or secondary tumor. Early detection is critical for treatment results.

This case is presented to remind people that persistent pain, unexplained weight loss, or worsening motor strength, balance or sensation must be evaluated fully.

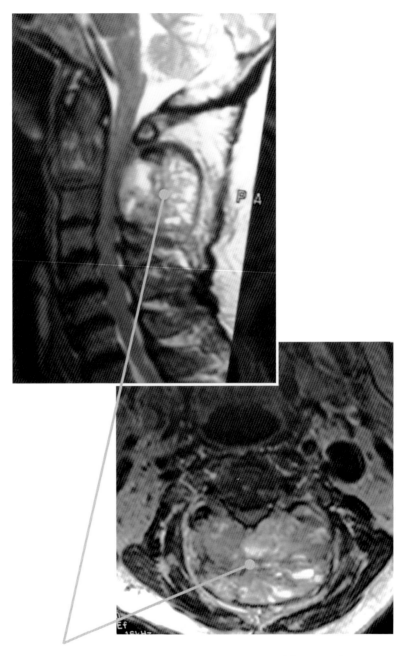

Large cervical mass involving the posterior aspect of the cervical spine
and causing spinal cord compression

CERVICAL FRACTURE

WITH ACTIVITIES, fractures about the cervical spine could occur. Patients complain of pain, stiffness and loss of range of motion. Sometimes paralysis might be present.

This gentleman was traveling in another country. He fell as he hopped cement blocks to stay out of high grass. The arrow shows the fracture of the lateral mass.

Despite long-standing conservative treatments, he had persistent pain requiring surgical stabilization with instrument fixation.

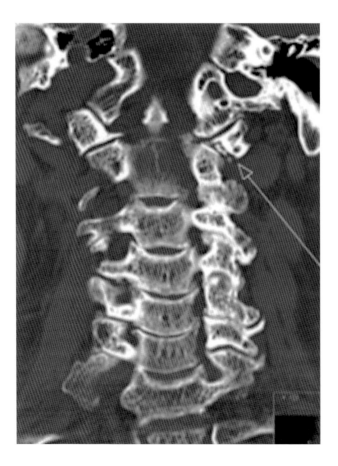

CHAPTER 4

Making The Diagnosis

HISTORY »
HIS OR HER STORY

A PHYSICIAN will sit down with a patient to gather a complete and focused history in an organized fashion, appropriate to the clinical situation. The goal is to understand the symptoms, level of suffering and what, if anything, has been done about it prior to that point. Patients typically complain of a sharp, lancing pain that progresses distally from the neck through the scapula, or shoulder blade, and into the various specific zones of the arm or hand. This is known as radiculopathy, a condition due to a compressed or irritated nerve in the spine that can cause pain, numbness, tingling, or weakness along the course of the nerve.

Nerves are very sophisticated "cables" in the body that transport information about pain, numbness, weakness, reflex changes, placement of an extremity in space, touch and feeling, fine point discrimination, and temperature. The type of symptoms that are experienced will determine which cables are compromised.

HISTORY OF PRESENT ILLNESS

How long has this been going on ?

What treatments did you try so far?

How successful were these treatments?

You will be asked to rate your pain

___/10 Neck   ___/10 Right Arm   ___/10 Left Arm

___/10 Back   ___/10 Right Leg   ___/10 Left Leg

Pain Rating System

0 = no pain

10 = worst possible pain

On the other hand, referred pain follows a non nerve and, therefore, nonspecific pattern. This tends to be a deeper and piercing pain.

Cauda equina syndrome, a condition where there is a compression of the nerves at the end of the spinal cord within the spinal canal, might exist with the onset of a loss of bowel/bladder control. This is usually a surgical emergency. Cauda equina could cause numbness of the genitalia (saddle anesthesia of the groin) and in both legs. **In this instance, go straight to your physician or the emergency room for immediate medical attention.** This could signify a compression of the nerves that innervate the bowel and bladder. When surgery is indicated, the best outcomes typically occur if surgical release is carried out within 6 hours of the onset of symptoms.

TYPICAL QUESTIONS ASKED BY THE PHYSICIAN

Numbness is the loss of sensation, usually of the arms and legs. Do you have any numbness?

Weakness is the loss of power of the arms and legs. Do you have any weakness?

Are there any functional losses, especially during activities of daily living?

+ A patient might note an inability to write properly, carry objects, throw a ball, or even brush their teeth or dress themselves.

I saw one of my patients in consult for a herniated disc. He kept his hand over his head for a year to relieve the pain. Surgical decompression was carried out. He has fully returned to all his activities and no longer needs to raise his hand over his head for temporary pain relief.

Bowel and bladder function are critical in spinal evaluation.

> ## RED FLAGS = TROUBLE
>
> A history of trauma suggests a fracture.
>
> Fever & chills may suggest an infection.
>
> Night Pain may suggest a tumor.
>
> Weight Loss may suggest a tumor.
>
> Loss of bowel and/or bladder control suggests myleopathy or a Cauda Equina Syndrome. Seek immediate medical treatment. There is typically a 6 hour window for emergency surgery, for the probable best outcome.

Examples of questions in regard to bowel function:

+ Do you have normal anal sensation?
+ Do you have good start and stop control?
+ Is there a history of bowel problems such as ulcerative colitis, Crohn's disease or other gastrointestinal problems?

Examples of questions in regard to bladder function:

+ Do you have any numbness of the genitalia area?
  + Numbness and power loss of the bladder is a serious emergency. Seek immediate medical attention.
+ Are you able to start and stop your urine flow with good control?
  + Some men with enlarged prostates have difficulty with starting or maintaining a stream.
  + Some women can naturally experience some leakage due to factors such as aging and cases of prolapse.

PHYSICAL EXAMINATION

PREVIOUS MEDICAL HISTORY

For a patient's personal safety, in regard to treatment options, the physician will assess for a history of medical problems. For example:

+ Diabetes
+ Hypertension
+ Heart Disease
+ Arterial Disease

PREVIOUS SPINAL SURGERY HISTORY
PREVIOUS SURGERY HISTORY

A patient should discuss any past spinal surgeries when seeing a physician that is not familiar with their history. They should be ready to explain the reasons for the operation, the name of the operation, the name of the surgeon, and how the operation has or has not benefitted them.

After any operation it is important that a personal copy of the records are kept, i.e. consults, imaging studies, MRIs, and X-rays. This will ensure that another physician or surgeon can properly resume patient care.

Similarly, patients should be ready to list and discuss any other type of previous surgeries that they have undergone. This is important information for the physician so a proper assessment, conclusion, and treatment plan can be made.

MEDICATIONS

Patients should be prepared to write a full list of the medications they are taking as well as past medications. Dosage, frequency, duration, and the physician that prescribed it is to be included.

Medication Name	Dosage	Frequency	How long have you taken this medication?	Prescribed by?

ALLERGIES

List all present and past allergies, and note the reaction to the allergy.

Allergy to	Type of Reaction

SOCIAL HISTORY

Do you smoke? If yes, how much?   How many years?

Do you drink? If yes, how much?   How many years?

Do you use illicit drugs? If yes, how much?   How many years?

The social history attempts to identify an individual's usage of cigarettes, alcohol, and illicit drugs.

PHYSICAL EXAMINATION

As spine specialists, we are trained to identify the compressed zones of the nerves. We most commonly identify the motor power function, the sensation distribution, and the reflex changes of each nerve. Typically, we are able to identify the nerve, or nerves, involved without an MRI scan.

The following diagrams will give you a better understanding of how we determine which nerve zone is compressed and also the way we, as spine specialists, think.

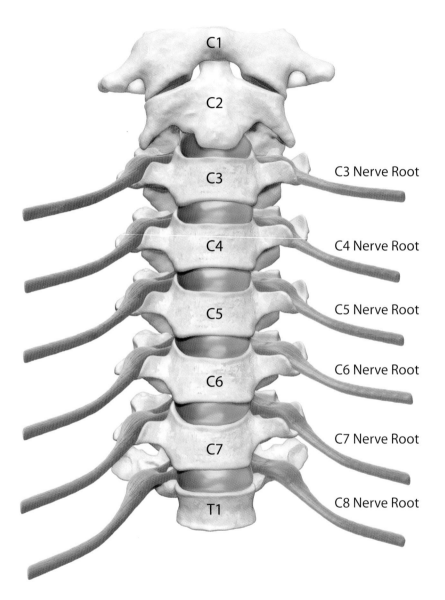

FRONT (ANTERIOR) VIEW
OF THE CERVICAL SPINE

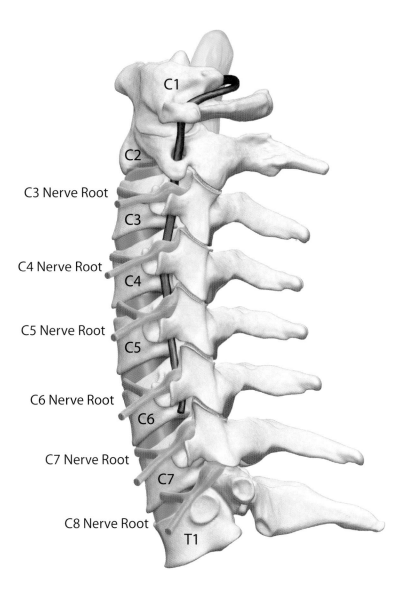

C1

C2

C3 Nerve Root

C3

C4 Nerve Root

C4

C5 Nerve Root

C5

C6 Nerve Root

C6

C7 Nerve Root

C7

C8 Nerve Root

T1

SIDE (LATERAL) VIEW
OF THE CERVICAL SPINE

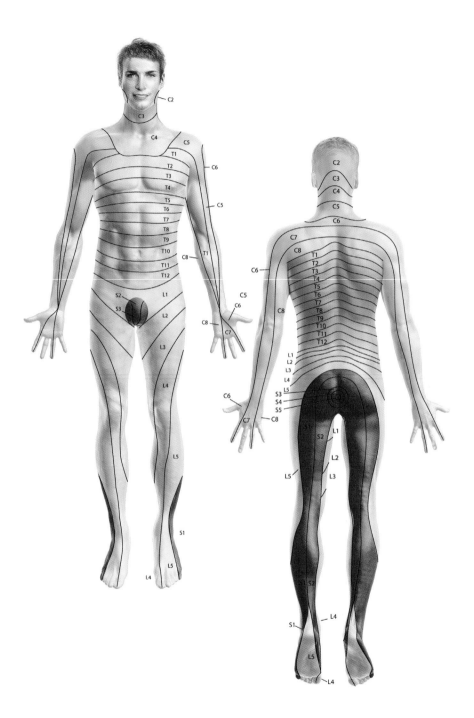

SENSORY ZONES

The body's sensory zones and zones of the ability to feel are shown in this diagram with the arrangement or distribution of nerves to an organ or body part (innervation).

The green-colored area represents the exit of the cervical spinal nerves from the neck and their innervation of the sensory zones.

The blue-colored area represents the exit of the thoracic spinal nerves from the thoracic spine and their innervation of the sensory zones.

The yellow-colored area represents the exit of the lumbar spinal nerves from the lumbar spine and their innervation of the sensory zones.

The red-colored area represents the exit of the sacral spinal nerves from the sacral spine and their innervation of the sensory and numbered levels zones.

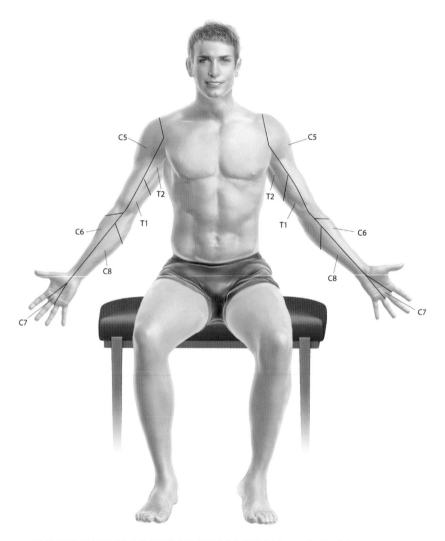

INNERVATION OF THE SENSORY ZONES OF THE ARM

C5 nerve = The outside portion of the arm

C6 nerve = The outside portion of the forearm and hand (thumb and index fingers)

C7 nerve = The middle finger

C8 nerve = The ring and little finger

T1 nerve = The inside of the arm - lower

T2 nerve = The inside of the arm - higher

C4–C5 DISC INTERSPACE CARRIES THE C5 NERVE ROOT

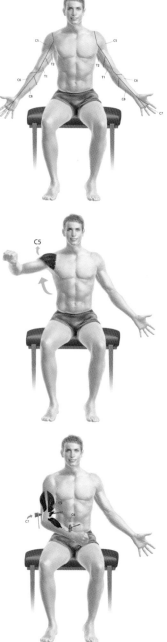

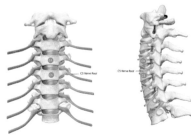

SENSATION

C5 supplies sensory innervation to the outside portion of the arm.

MOTOR

The deltoid muscle, which elevates the arm, is at the level of the shoulder.

REFLEX

The biceps reflex carries both C5 and C6 information.

C5–C6 DISC INTERSPACE CARRIES THE C6 NERVE ROOT

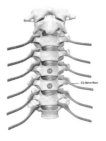
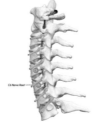

SENSATION
C6 supplies sensory innervation to the outside portion of the forearm and hand (thumb and index fingers)

MOTOR
The biceps and brachioradialis, depicted in the right arm, have C6 innervation. The wrist extensor muscle, depicted in the left wrist, allows extension of the wrist.

REFLEX
The brachioradialis reflex (shown in the right forearm) carries C6 information.

C6 – C7 DISC INTERSPACE CARRIES THE
C7 NERVE ROOT

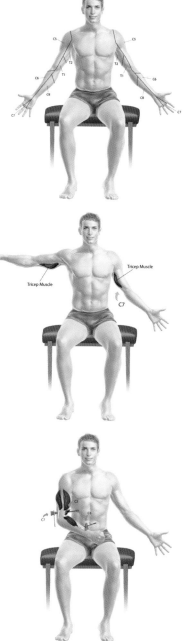

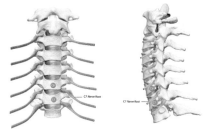

SENSATION
C7 supplies sensory innervation to the middle finger.

MOTOR
The triceps muscle depicted on both arms, and the wrist flexor depicted on the right wrist, have C7 innervation.

REFLEX
The triceps reflex carries predominantly C7 information.

C7–T1 DISC INTERSPACE CARRIES THE C8 NERVE ROOT

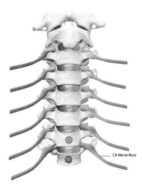 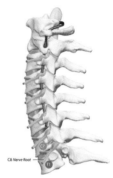

SENSATION

C8 supplies sensory innervation to the inner portion of the forearm and the ring and little finger.

MOTOR

The wrist flexor muscles are important in grip strength.

*Reflex: there is no reflex that carries discrete C8 information.

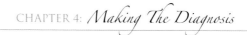

T1 – T2 DISC INTERSPACE CARRIES THE T1 NERVE ROOT

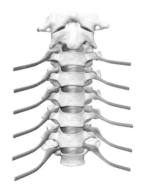
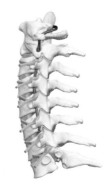

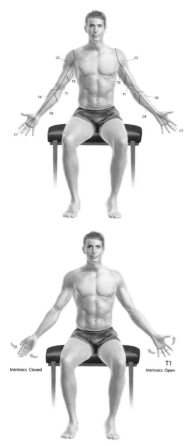

SENSATION

T1 supplies sensory innervation to the inner portion of the lower arm.

*Reflex: there is no reflex that carries discrete T1 information.

MOTOR

The fine intrinsic muscles (those originating at the wrist and within the hand) are important for grip. The right hand shows the fingers are being closed with the use of the intrinsic muscles. The left hand shows the fingers are being opened with the use of the intrinsic muscles.

IMAGING EVALUATION

WITH MODERN DAY imaging services, we can see more accurately and precisely. Indeed, a visit to a spine specialist without an imaging study could be considered a social visit.

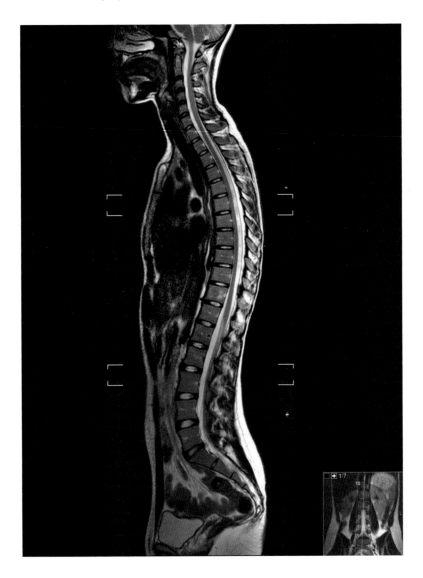

X-RAY FINDINGS

X-rays are necessary to identify the bones, bony alignment and general outline of the spinal canal.

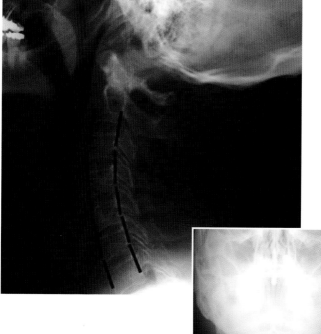

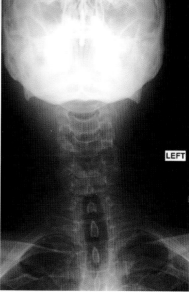

Standard X-rays show the bone quality and structure. Alignment of the columns of spinal bones are clearly shown.

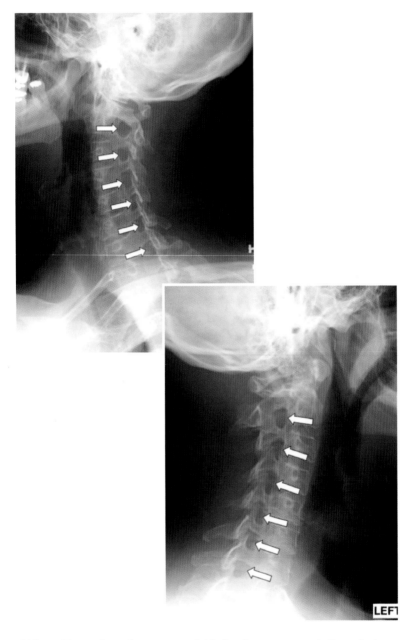

Oblique X-rays show the spaces available for the nerves to exit from the bony channels, called the neuroforamen. Views of the left and right neuroforamen are usually taken.

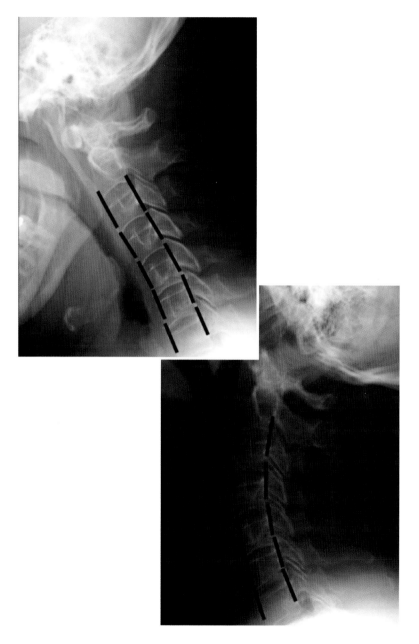

Flexion view (on the left) and extension view (on the right) are techniques used to assess for motion of the vertebral bodies.

MAGNETIC RESONANCE IMAGING

MRI really defines and shows the soft tissue of the spinal canal (spinal cord, nerve roots, and ligaments).

Bony landmarks are also shown with an MRI.

Diseases involving the bones are identified using various enhancement techniques. While common causes such as herniation, stenosis, and degenerative disc disease are the most common findings, infections of the bone and disc could also be identified as well as tumors.

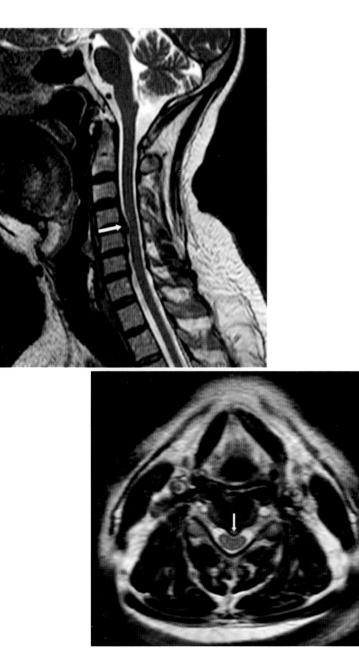

A sagittal (side) view and an axial (sliced) view show a centrally herniated disc at the C4–C5 interspace level.

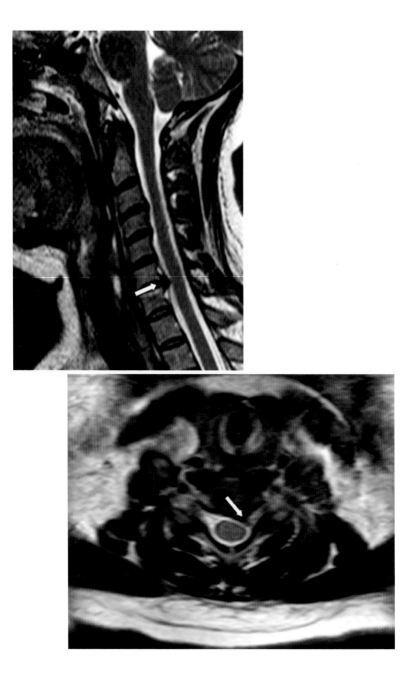

A sagittal (side) view and an axial (sliced) view show a left sided herniated disc at C6–C7.

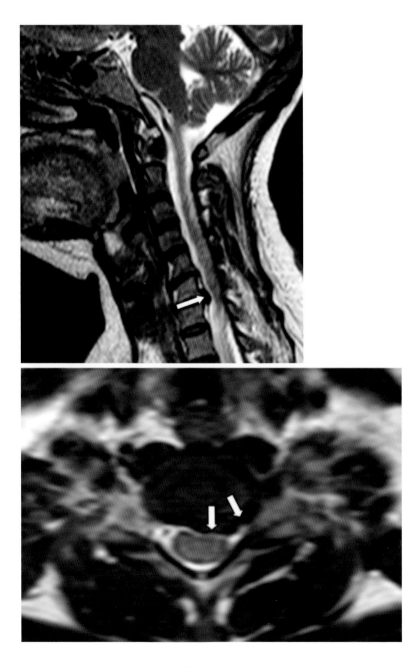

A sagittal (side) view and an axial (sliced) view show compression of the spinal elements from cervical stenosis.

MYELOPATHY

Myelopathy refers to the compression of the spinal cord to the extent that it is visibly swollen. A physical examination could show spastic weakness and greater weakness in the upper body. When ambulatory, the patient might display a broad-based shuffling gate due to the loss of the ability to coordinate muscular movement (ataxia). Incoordination might be present in one or both limbs.

Lhermitte's sign, an electrical or lighting-like sensation that runs down the back and into the limbs when bending the head forward, might be present. It is otherwise described as electrical shocks with a burning sensation in the trunks or limbs, usually caused by flexion of the neck.

It is possible to observe changes in anal sphincter function. Similarly, it is possible for urinary retention to occur.

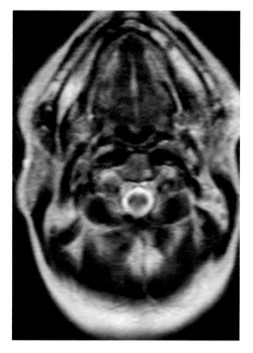

NORMAL SPINAL CORD
Spinal fluid is seen around the spinal cord.

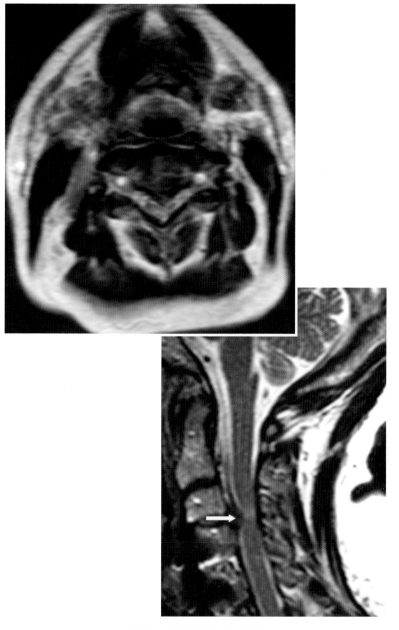

COMPRESSED CORD
No fluid is seen. White area within spinal cord = myelomalacia
or spinal cord swelling

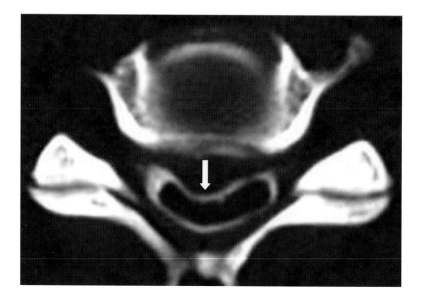

A CT-Myelogram is an invasive study using the placement of dye. This technique is used, for example, when an MRI is not possible in a patient with an implanted pacemaker. In this image, a large herniation is shown in the neck.

Case supplied by Dr. Leslie Saint-Louis of New York City.

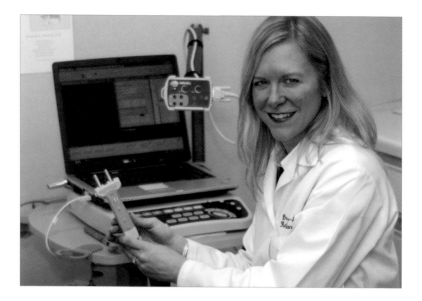

EMG ASSESSMENTS

Electromyography (EMG) is a form of electro-diagnostic testing that is used to study nerve and muscle function.

This test is usually performed by a physical medicine and rehabilitation specialist or a neurologist that is trained in this procedure. EMG testing can provide your doctor with specific information about the extent of a nerve and/or muscle injury. It can also determine the precise location of the injury and provide some indication whether or not the damage is reversible.

Occasionally, when there are many levels of compression, we use an EMG to assess, electrically, which nerve roots are symptomatic. Some nerve roots can be compressed but not symptomatic. This allows us to develop strategies to perform more limited surgical operations.

CHAPTER 5

Human Software

IMPORTANCE OF THINKING
MEDITATION
POSITIVE PSYCHOLOGY
POSITIVE/NEGATIVE THOUGHT
NEUROPLASTICITY
AMYGDALA PLASTICITY
SILENCE, SOLITUDE, STILLNESS
& HAPPINESS

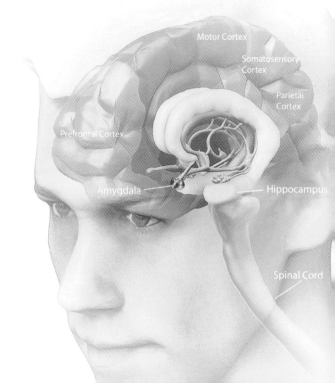

IMPORTANCE OF THINKING

PEOPLE EVERYWHERE are suffering. Spinal problems are global in nature and the damage to humanity goes beyond the physical well-being. In the United States alone, the cost of spinal conservative options and surgeries have reached an astronomical height of $100 billion annually.

Many of my clients are fascinated with spinal technology and the advances made in the field, which are helpful to all parties involved when spinal surgery is needed and employed.

The next two chapters introduce "six physicians": Sun, Air, Water, Diet, Exercise and Rest. Techniques are described which are available to everyone in their day to day life. These approaches are intrinsic to the human condition and could easily be applied to a daily regimen with no additional expense.

Study them, understand them and use them everyday.

Insanity is doing the same thing over and over and expecting a different result.

Albert Einstein

Becoming a master is not about
doing 4,000 things.
It is about doing
12 things 4,000 times.

Chet Holmes

Successful people ask better questions,
and as a result,
they get better answers.

Anthony Robbins

INNER WORK –
HUMAN SOFTWARE
ASSESSMENT

T HE OUTER-MOST LAYERS of the physical self are manifested as the body with subsequent realizations of pleasure versus pain. Underneath is the inner layer, a virtual "software" recorded in the neurons of the brain and the nervous system manifested in the heart, the gut, and all the nerves. This, seemingly indefinable, ethereal layer is the most important. It is responsible for what drives people; it is more real and more sophisticated than the software in your computer.

So many people just live and work without ever taking the time to work on the software that acts as the body's control center. Very few are aware of the importance of the development of the inner layer in physical and mental well-being and even less are thoughtful enough to put in the time to do so.

Who am I? What are my identities? What do I stand for? These are a few examples of the questions presented above that have driven great philosophers and thinkers such as Socrates and Confucius. I recommend making many passes at these questions as often as possible. Each pass leads to a deeper answer and a deeper understanding of self.

INNER WORK	TODAY
Who am I?	
What are my identities?	
What do I stand for?	
What rules do I live by?	
What do I love?	
What do I hate?	
What excites me?	
What makes me happy?	
What am I committed to?	
What do I regret?	
What must I do before I die?	

THE POWER OF A POSITIVE THOUGHT, OR A RANDOM ACT OF KINDNESS

With a positive thought,
OR WITH A RANDOM ACT OF KINDNESS:

+ the brain is calm
+ the body moves into a rest and digest mode
+ there are fewer "pressors" (chemicals e.g. epinephrine, that raise the blood pressure)
+ the heart feels good
+ the body relaxes and takes breaths deep into the lungs
+ the intestines work on digestion more efficiently
+ libido is increased
+ muscles loosen and are more mobile
+ the arteries don't experience an excessive amount of pressors, creating a normotensive state (having normal blood pressure)
+ there are less inflammatory factors in your blood stream
+ the pancreas and thyroid function optimally
+ the immune system peaks, helping to ward off infection
+ inflammation decreases, increasing body resting and functioning
+ there is decreased tenderness and discomfort due to spinal problems

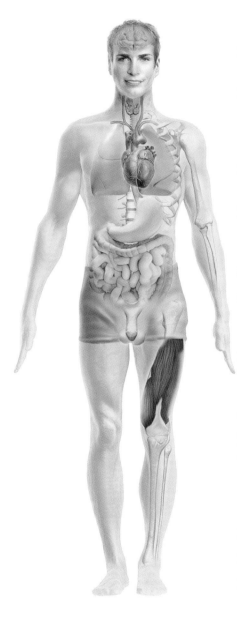

+ THOUGHT

Brain: Calm, possibly excited

Hormones: Thyroid, pancreas, liver etc. Optimal production and function

Lungs: Full, deep breathing

Heart: Feels good Regular beat and rhythm

Spinal Nerves: Not Inflamed

Spinal Facets: Flexible, not inflamed and best function

Nerves: Parasympathetic = body is resting and digesting

GI Tract: Rest and digest

Reproductive organs: + Libido Male: optimal testosterone Female: menstrual regularity

Muscles: Mobile, non-tender

Ligaments: Flexible

Bones: Ready for action

– THOUGHT

Brain:	Anxious, depression, restlessness
Hormones:	Thyroid, pancreas, liver, etc. Sub-optimal production and function
Lungs:	Shallow, irregular breathing
Heart:	Feels unsettled Irregular beat and rhythm
Spinal Nerves:	Inflamed with pain, numbness, and weakness
Spinal Facets:	Inflamed and diminished function
Nerves:	Sympathetic = body is getting ready for fight or flight
GI Tract:	Indigestion and ulcers
Reproductive organs:	Diminished Libido Male: decreased testosterone Female: menstrual irregularity
Muscles:	Stiff, tender
Ligaments:	Stiff
Bones:	Increased chance for injury

THE DANGERS OF A NEGATIVE THOUGHT

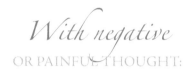

With negative
OR PAINFUL THOUGHT:

+ the brain is in turmoil
+ the body moves into fight or flight mode
+ there are more pressors
+ the heart develops an irregular rate and rhythm
+ stress increases and shallow breaths are taken into the lungs
+ digestion slows in the intestines and ulcers may develop from stress
+ reproductive hormones are affected and libido is decreased
+ muscles tighten and become more tender
+ the arteries experience excessive pressors, increasing the chance of hypertension
+ inflammatory factors in the blood stream increase, and irritability increases
+ the pancreas and thyroid do not function optimally, increasing blood sugar levels and thyroid hormone output to become dysfunctional
+ the immune system weakens, increasing risk of infection
+ there is a greater chance of tenderness and discomfort due to spinal problems

NEUROPLASTICITY

EVEN AS A PHYSICIAN, it was my thought that the brain was an ever-decaying organ. We are born with hundreds of billions of brain cells, of which most are not used. Toward the end of one's life there is a watershed area. Recently, there has been an emergence of a new thinking referred to as neuroplasticity (neuro = brain, plastic = changeable).

Backed by modern neurological science, neuroplasticity is the theory that as we perform acts and as we think, new tracks and connections are laid down in the brain. In other words, the brain becomes "wired."

Further wiring of the same tracts lead to thicker cortices, the outer layer of the cerebrum, which plays an important role in consciousness. The brain progresses into a master level of function after experiencing wiring for the same activity or skill for 10,000 hours (approximately 10 years). This trained brain is capable of "seeing" things that a less developed brain cannot.

Constructive Neuroplasticity: Purposeful and definitive thinking, and acting in those manners create neurons and define the brain tracks that constitute your brain. Imagination and visualizations also serve to build neurons.

Degenerative Neuroplasticity: Depressing and/or terrible thoughts and acting in a manner which wires the brain with a negative outlook.

People should be careful not to allow certain thoughts into the brain for prolonged periods of time and also take caution when choosing the activities in which they engage. Just as purposeful and definitive thinking can be wired into the brain, negative thinking can be also.

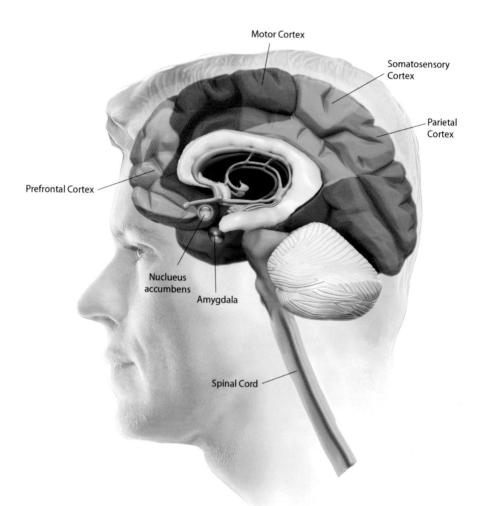

NEUROPLASTICITY AS EXPRESSED WITH ROBIN SHARMA'S EIGHT FORMS OF WEALTH

AUTHOR AND LEADERSHIP EXPERT Robin Sharma (www.RobinSharma.com) defined the eight forms of wealth. Sharma expressed that there are eight elements that you want to make sure are at world-class levels before you call yourself rich and truly successful. He defines them as inner life, physical wealth, family and social wealth, career wealth, economic wealth, circle of genius, adventure success, and impact wealth. This figure shows that with thinking and doing we build neurons that are developed with as much care, time and tendering that we spend in achieving the eight forms of wealth. This inner mental wiring matches our outer world wiring and performance. This inner hard wire could also be the basis of our conscience.

The inner and outer worlds are manifested about the body. Clinical research suggests that the vast majority of humans have definite nerve root compressions in the spine, but the majority are without symptoms. I propose that parts of spinal pain may be manifestations of inner world turmoil expressed as outer world pain.

The figure opposite is an illustration of a neuron for the purpose of depicting the eight forms of wealth.

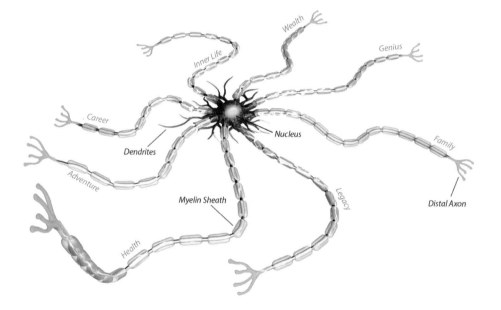

ROBIN SHARMA'S EIGHT FORMS OF WEALTH
Dramatization of a neuron for depiction purposes.

AMYGDALA
NEUROPLASTICITY

THE AMYGDALA is a well studied part of the brain due to its established role in memory, specific emotional responses, hormonal secretions and disorders such as fear, anxiety, depression, and autism. It is also part of the reptilian brain.

The brain processes signals by sending information through the thalamus to the neocortex which is better known as the thinking portion of the brain. From there, the neocortex forwards the signal to the amygdala or the emotional part of the brain.

Most human sequence of thought, emotion and action occur in this manner. Many emotions are driven by thought but not all. For example, when the brain perceives a potential threat the thalamus often bypasses the cortex and sends the signal directly to the amygdala, triggering what is better known as a "fight or flight" response. The amygdala responds with immediate emotion, which causes specific physical changes. For example, senses sharpen, the cardio-vascular and respiratory systems jump into action, fat from fatty cells and glucose from the liver are metabolized for instant energy, blood vessels constrict to shut down non-essential systems and to reduce any potential blood loss, endorphins are released as a natural pain killer, and the natural judgment system is turned down and more primitive responses take over.

In his book *Emotional Intelligence: Why It Can Matter More Than IQ*, Daniel Golean defines the term "Amygdala Hijack" to describe emotional responses from people that are out of measure with the actual threat. The hijack occurs when the frontal cortex is bypassed and decisions are made primarily from the amygdala.

Studies have revealed that the amygdala is a complex and dynamic brain region that serves as the "Grand Central Station" for emotions. The

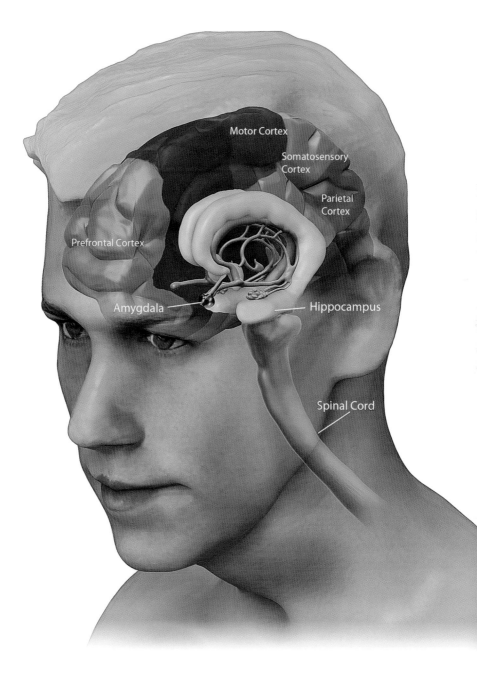

literature makes it clear that non-neuronal glial cells, sometimes called the neuroglia or simply glia, in the amygdala are sensitive and plastic cells that respond and develop in a highly region-specific manner.

Harvard psychologist, Britta Holzel, and her colleagues published a controlled longitudinal study to investigate pre- and post-changes in brain gray matter concentration attributable to participation using Mindfulness-Based Stress Reduction (MBSR). One of the most widely recognized programs of its type, MBSR has been shown to produce positive effects on psychological well-being and to improve symptoms of a number of disorders.

An eight-week MBSR program involved before and after anatomical Magnetic Resonance Images (MRI) from 16 healthy participants introduced to meditation and a control group of 17 individuals that did not practice meditation. Any changes in gray matter concentration of the two groups were recorded using voxel-based morphometry, a neuroimaging analysis technique that allows investigation of focal differences in brain anatomy. Analysis of MRI brain scans taken after the participants' meditation regimen found increased gray matter in the hippocampus, an area in the brain that is important for learning and memory. Images of the meditation group also showed a reduction of gray matter in the amygdala. The control group did not show such changes.

Why does a spinal surgeon write so enthusiastically about the amygdala? It is now well known that the brain is plastic. The ability for scientists to identify the plasticity of the amygdala, the critical emotional Grand Central Station of the brain, is the fundamental basis for true hope. Thoughts and the usual emotions are the basis for all our actions in our body and self. Spinal health is one result of great thoughts, emotions and actions.

I believe that future research could show that the deeply depressed person or the alcoholic could expect transformation and plastic changes in the origin of emotions. There is a direct relationship of depression and alcoholic neuropathy to spinal nerve pain.

There are enough cases of people who self-medicated with alcohol because it feels better when, indeed, there is a structural source of pain such as spinal stenosis or hip arthritis.

MEDITATION

MEDITATION IS THE PROCESS of calming the body and mind while allowing a connection with the universe. We are all so busy with our day to day activities and thoughts that we lose track of our goals, our vision, and our life plan. This non-stop grind prevents us from being thoughtful and performing the tasks necessary for our well-being and body maintenance.

Traditional Meditation involves sitting in a quiet, calm and peaceful place. My mother taught me to keep my spine straight and to breathe in and out with intention as I sat in a cross-legged sitting posture, known as the lotus position, that originated in meditative practices of ancient India.

Deeper meditation such as alternate nostril breathing includes breathing through one nostril at a time and out through the opposite. Yogis believe that this exercise will cleanse and rejuvenate your vital channels of energy. As you sit, thoughts, emotions, and feelings will come to you. Recognize them and allow them to pass without letting yourself become attached. The thoughts and emotions diminish with time, which allows access to universal thoughts and energies. This process is great for resetting our minds from the frustrations and negativity that prevent us from achieving our daily regimens that keep us healthy and pain free. Today could be the start of your great new world. Learning how to meditate could easily be searched on www.youtube.com

Guided Imagery is the process of sitting in a quiet, comfortable place while relaxing and following audio or video instructions. An instructor guides you through various scenarios of directed thoughts and suggestions that lead your imagination toward a relaxed, focused state to help cleanse physical and emotional burdens. Free guided imagery sequences are easily found with an Internet search. I'm a fan of "Meditation for Elite Performers," which can be downloaded at www.RobinSharma.com.

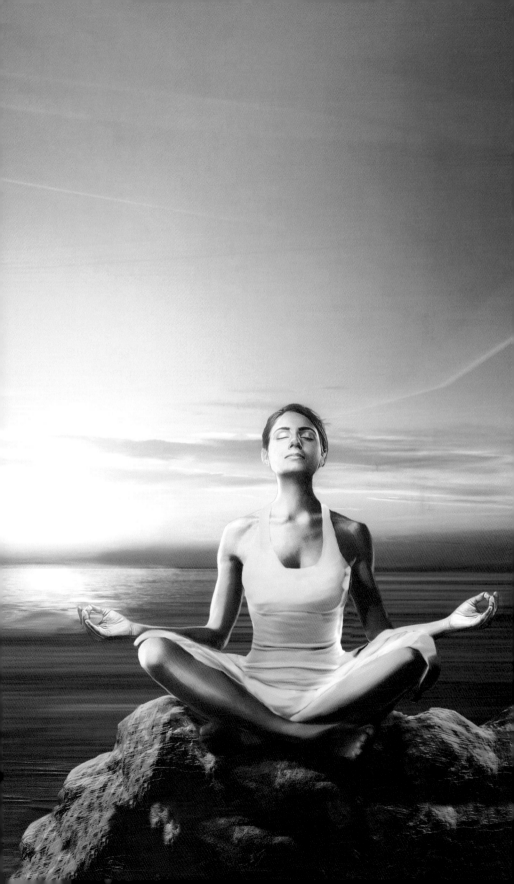

HYPNOSIS

Hypnosis is the strategy of placing suggestions through the conscious mind to the subconscious mind. John Assaraf, author of *The Answer* has developed a program combining meditation, affirmations, brain entrainment and hypnosis for business people. Learn more about this at www.johnassaraf.com.

BRAIN-WAVE ENTRAINMENT

Properly engineered brainwave entrainment uses deeply relaxing sound recordings, known as isochronic or monaural tones, to pulse your neurons at specific frequencies to put the listener into a similar state reached through disciplined meditation typically achieved by Zen masters.

Internationally recognized brain-wave entrainment engineer, Morry Zelcovitch advised me that with an optimized brain it is easy to improve sleep, reduce stress, increase personal happiness and health, and diminish pain. More information on this subject can be found at www.quantum-mind-power.com. Morry's group is currently developing elite optimizations for soldiers and extreme athletes.

The figure to the right shows that tones and strategies can be developed to diminish the wave-lengths of the left sided "thinking and worrying" brain. At the same time tones and strategies may be used to amplify the right "creative" brain. If it is necessary to amplify the logical, thinking brain and diminish the creative urges, then reverse the headset.

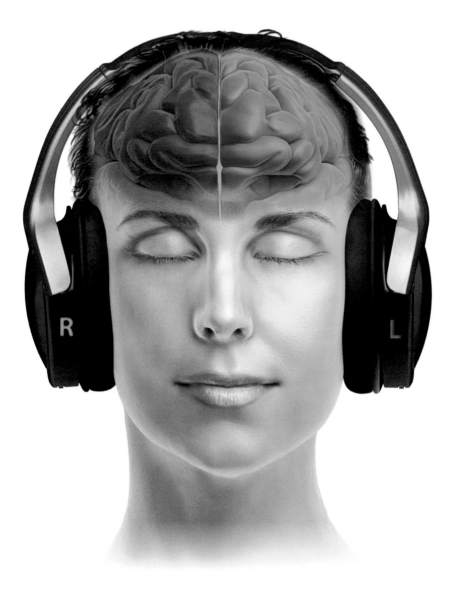

SILENCE, SOLITUDE & STILLNESS

MODERN DAY LIVING leads us to do more, say more, drive more, and work longer, harder and faster. The tendency is to eat poorly and quickly, drive quickly, work quickly, play less, rest less, sleep less and wake earlier. The pressure of go, go, go leads to a vicious cycle of not resting, eating, sleeping and recuperating. Finally, there's a loss of productivity in our personal and professional life.

Planning time out daily for silence, solitude and stillness allows us to break the cycle. The goal is to be thoughtful with our words and actions and to plan our lives and make healthy, productive choices. This will help our spine and nerves stay or become healthy.

HAPPINESS

Most folks are about as happy as they make their minds up to be.

Abraham Lincoln

INTERNAL HAPPINESS

Spinal health is integrally related to emotional health and happiness. With positive emotional health, the same spinal nerve, with a bit of stenosis or compression, or the mildly arthritic facet joint has the best chance of being pain-free.

With diminished emotional health, the same spinal nerve with a bit of stenosis or compression, or the mildly arthritic facet joint has the least chance of being pain-free.

As a physician working on defining happiness, this process of producing a "happy person" begins with an understanding of our human body's parts, structures and functions. I believe that it is easier to achieve happiness by embracing physical fitness.

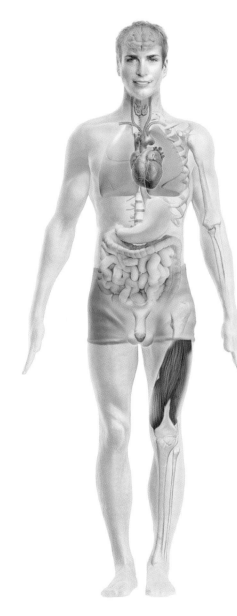

Brain: Function and especially thoughts

Carotid artery: An indicator of the health of multiple systems in the body

Thyroid: Hormone driver

Heart health: Studies show that the heart and spinal health are linked

Lungs health: Every breath you take is important. As you breathe the spinal nerves move in the spinal canal

Gastro-intestinal tract: Carries tremendous implications of diet, hormones, stress factors and immunity

Genitourinal tract: Emphasis on hormone metabolism and sexual health

Muscle health: A good layer of functional muscles is important for physical performance and emotional well-being

Bone health: Great bones are made by paying attention to calcium and vitamin D intake, the pounding of weight-bearing exercise, and strength training.

EXTERNAL HAPPINESS

The emerging field of positivity identifies commitment to work, genetics, relationships, spirituality, certain foods, intention, choices, a happy marriage, finances, gratitude, volunteering, random acts of kindness and of less importance, money, home, car and a high position as important factors that drive external happiness.

I believe and feel that awareness of the physical body, exercise and body construction is one the most important drivers of external happiness. I have used the concepts of aerobic, plyometric and strength training with the use of yoga techniques as a mode of personal physical transformation.

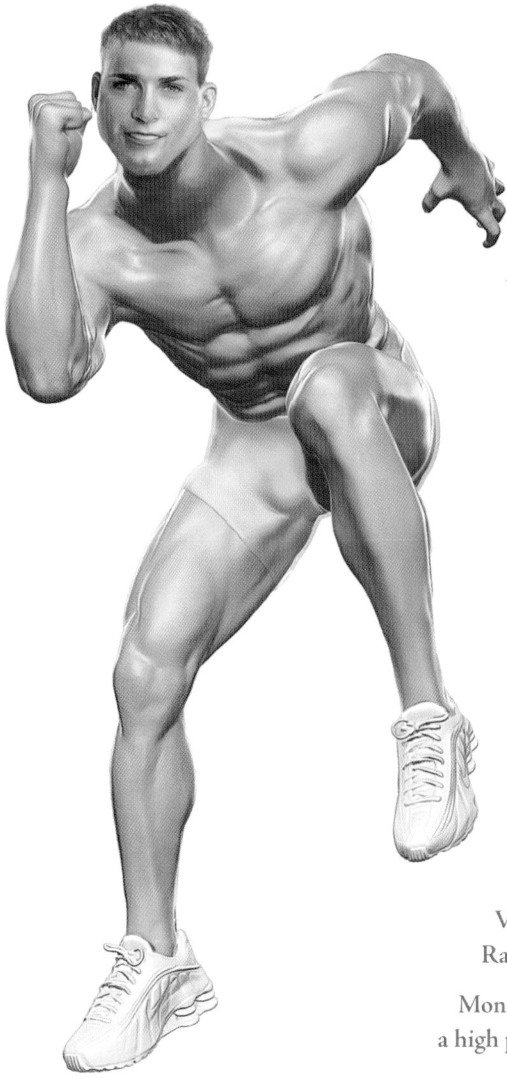

Work aka flow

Gratitude

A happy marriage

Relationships with
friends and family

50% Genetics

Spirituality

Chocolates & apples

Smiling

Ha Ha He He exercises

Finances

Intention & Choice

Physical fitness

Volunteering/
Random acts of kindness

Money, home, car, and
a high position

POSITIVE PSYCHOLOGY

TRADITIONAL PSYCHOLOGY focuses on what made us dysfunctional, ill, or depressed. Summed up in 1998, a branch of the mental health field known as positive psychology has emerged to complement, not to replace, traditional psychology. Positive psychology is a study of the strengths and virtues that enable individuals and communities to thrive. Institutes such as the Positive Psychology Center at the University of Pennsylvania focus on mental wellness with the implementation of three central concerns: positive emotions, positive individual traits, and positive institutions. Prominent among the field is Dr. Martin Seligman, director of the Positive Psychology Center. Seligman is known for focusing on and defining what can go right.

Hungarian psychology professor Mihaly Csikszentmihalyi wrote the classic paper, "Flow: The Psychology of Optimal Experience." Csikszentmihalyi's theory states that people are most happy when they are in a mode of concentration or complete absorption with the activity at hand, otherwise known as "flow." The whole being is involved and the ego and any self gratifying needs dissipate. This ideology can be traced back to prominent historical figures such as Michelangelo who had a deep spiritual conviction and was inspired by a life that had meaning. His recommendation is to be in love with what you do.

A review of the National Library of Medicine's world's literature on positivity is remarkable. The authors were amazed with the findings that connected happiness to physical well-being. Put simply, the studies showed that happy people become more satisfied due to the fact that they develop resources for living well. Strategies to engage and stimulate these people improved their sense of well-being, happiness, and general health.

In 1996, University of Minnesota research scientist David Lykken looked at the role of genes in determining one's sense of satisfaction in life. Lykken studied 4,000 sets of twins born in Minnesota from 1936 to 1955. After comparing identical and fraternal twins happiness data, he concluded that about 50% of an individual's satisfaction with life is due to genetic programming. Lykken reported that factors like income, marital status, religion, and education contribute approximately only 8 percent to overall well-being.

Some people are taught from a young age that money, home, car, and a high position and stature in life are important factors in developing a sense of high self-esteem. However, studies show that the effect of income on life satisfaction seems to be transient. It is being in a happy marriage that has been directly associated with overall well-being and health benefits such as lower morbidity and mortality.

Breathing could change in response to sadness, happiness, anxiety, or fear. One paper concluded that "our results indicate that what is really important is not what one has but how he sees, evaluates, and experiences what he has." Another study summarized that "the person's level of consciousness and responsible attitude toward life and others seem far more important for the global quality of life and health."

Happiness begins with your thoughts. Most times we are not aware of where we are in the spectrum of living. It is easy to think, "Oh, I wish I had a better job, better car, and a more appreciative family." People postpone their happiness while they work to build a better career, a better body, or a better position in life. Once an elevated position or stature is achieved, often times people find that they are less happy than before they made those changes. Brainwave entrainment engineer Morry Zelcovitch recommends to cut to the chase, skip the steps of development and choose to be happy, NOW!

Genetics tries to hold individuals to a happiness set point. This might be a higher point of happiness than is currently being experienced. Life's dedication to work and profession, which is an example of flow, is the main driver to happiness. There are other drivers within one's power that could be responsible for the critical 1% that propels them into absolute happiness. Nevertheless, I fully recognize that sadness and depression has a role in our human experience, just as winter has a place among the seasons.

Scientists Chida and Steptoe showed that anger and hostility are associated with coronary heart disease in both patients suffering from heart disease and healthy people.

Happiness is a state of mind that can be planned, influenced, and accomplished; it is a choice. Set a definite intention and choose to be happy today. Achievement of happiness may benefit from meditations on personal thoughts, actions, gratitude, and intentions. Be committed to the process and test yourself throughout the day. Journal your experiences daily.

Significant happiness could be derived from being grateful for all that one has as well as from family, friends, and organizations, etc. with which they are associated. People that give to charity, for example, are associated with healthier and happier lives. Taking the time to be grateful, thankful and thoughtful could help develop an appreciation of the true wealth of life. Author Borgonovi showed that volunteering leads to happiness.

Optimism investigators Diener and Seligman opined that the most salient characteristics shared by students, with the highest levels of happiness and the fewest signs of depression, were their strong ties to friends and family and the commitment to spending time with them.

Studies show that foods such as chocolate and apples might elevate mood. Not surprisingly, chocolate seems to be the more strongly perceived mood elevator by most people. I specifically recommend savoring chocolates, but if you are eating for hunger choose the apple.

Regular exercise and fitness performed with a flow component has helped me achieve, significantly, elevated levels of mood and happiness.

Smile as much as you can. The muscles of the mouth can be used in a conscious attempt to smile and be happy. My staff and I do the ha ha, he he exercises! Break into two groups and try it.

Group 1: Ha ha ha ha ha ha!   **Group 2: He he he he he he!**

When you are happy the brain has a particular chemistry of serotonins which are biochemically derived from tryptophan and a known contributor to well-being, catecholamines which are fight or flight hormones released by the adrenal glands, norepinephrine, and dopamine. When dopamine or norepinephrine is produced, we tend to act and think more quickly and are generally more alert. Complex carbohydrates raise levels of tryptophan in the brain and have a calming effect. Proteins promote the production of dopamine and norepinephrine which promote alertness.

AFFIRMATIONS

AN AFFIRMATION is a declaration that something is true. As we go through our day, we are constantly thinking and sending ourselves various messages known as self-talk.

New neural plasticity science is saying that whatever a person thinks becomes wired into the neurons of the brain. With constant repetition these thoughts fire neurons which generate tracks and, subsequently, become embedded permanently in the brain. It is at this level of "thought" that we, as humans, write the software that becomes embedded in our minds and that run our lives. Thoughts become emotions, then emotions manifest actions, which generate the pieces of one's life.

SELF-TALK CAN BE POSITIVE:

"I'm a good person, doing good things for people."
"I'm improving myself in every way each day."
"I'm awesome."
"I'm good enough, I'm smart enough, and people like me."

SELF-TALK CAN BE NEGATIVE:

"I'm a loser."
"I never do much anyway."
"My life is a waste."

BIBLIOGRAPHY

THE POWER OF A POSITIVE THOUGHT, OR A RANDOM ACT OF KINDNESS

Abboud FM. *Physiology in perspective: The wisdom of the body. In search of autonomic balance: the good, the bad, and the ugly.* The Walter B. Cannon Memorial Award Lecture, 2009. Am J Physiol Regul Integr Comp Physiol. 2010 Jun;298(6):R1449-67. Epub 2010 Mar 10.

Dhalla NS, Adameova A, Kaur M. *Role of catecholamine oxidation in sudden cardiac death.* Fundam Clin Pharmacol. 2010 Oct;24(5):539-46. doi: 10.1111/j.1472-8206.2010.00836.x.

Dünser MW, Hasibeder WR. *Sympathetic overstimulation during critical illness: adverse effects of adrenergic stress.* J Intensive Care Med. 2009 Sep-Oct;24(5):293-316. Epub 2009 Aug 23.

Giacco F, Brownlee M. *Oxidative stress and diabetic complications.* Circ Res. 2010 Oct 29;107(9):1058-70. Diabetes Research Center, Departments of Medicine/Endocrinology, Albert Einstein College of Medicine, 1300 Morris Park Ave., Bronx, New York 10461-1602, USA.

Kalsbeek A, Bruinstroop E, Yi CX, Klieverik LP, La Fleur SE, Fliers E. *Hypothalamic control of energy metabolism via the autonomic nervous system.* Ann N Y Acad Sci. 2010 Nov;1212:114-29. doi: 10.1111/j.1749-6632.2010.05800.x. Epub 2010 Nov 11.

Lewis KS, Whipple JK, Michael KA, Quebbeman EJ. *Effect of analgesic treatment on the physiological consequences of acute pain.* Am J Hosp Pharm. 1994 Jun 15;51(12):1539-54.

Low CA, Thurston RC, Matthews KA. *Psychosocial factors in the development of heart disease in women: current research and future directions.* Psychosom Med. 2010 Nov;72(9):842-54. Epub 2010 Sep 14.

Navarro X. *Physiology of the autonomic nervous system.* Rev Neurol. 2002 Sep 16-30;35(6):553-62.

Otaka M, Odashima M, Tamaki K, Watanabe S. *Expression and function of stress (heat shock) proteins in gastrointestinal tract.* Int J Hyperthermia. 2009 Dec;25(8):634-40.

Pitocco D, Zaccardi F, Di Stasio E, Romitelli F, Santini SA, Zuppi C, Ghirlanda G. *Oxidative stress, nitric oxide, and diabetes.* Rev Diabet Stud. 2010 Spring;7(1):15-25. Epub 2010 May 10.

Qin W, Bauman WA, Cardozo CP. *Evolving concepts in neurogenic osteoporosis.* Curr Osteoporos Rep. 2010 Dec;8(4):212-8.

Radley JJ, Morrison JH. *Repeated stress and structural plasticity in the brain.* Ageing Res Rev. 2005 May;4(2):271-87.

Roberts CK, Sindhu KK. *Oxidative stress and metabolic syndrome.* Life Sci. 2009 May 22;84(21-22):705-12. Epub 2009 Mar 9.

Roozendaal B, McEwen BS, Chattarji S. *Stress, memory and the amygdala.* Nat Rev Neurosci. 2009 Jun;10(6):423-33. Department of Neuroscience, University Medical Center Groningen, University of Groningen, the Netherlands. b.roozendaal@med.umcg.nl

Schömig A, Richardt G, Kurz T. *Sympatho-adrenergic activation of the ischemic myocardium and its arrhythmogenic impact.* Herz. 1995 Jun;20(3):169-86.

Schömig A, Richardt G. *The role of catecholamines in ischemia.* J Cardiovasc Pharmacol. 1990;16 Suppl 5:S105-12.

Thorsell A. *Brain neuropeptide Y and corticotropin-releasing hormone in mediating stress and anxiety.* Exp Biol Med (Maywood). 2010 Oct 1;235(10):1163-7.

West NP, Pyne DB, Peake JM, Cripps AW. *Probiotics, immunity and exercise: a review.* Exerc Immunol Rev. 2009;15:107-26.

NEUROPLASTICITY

Radley JJ, Morrison JH. *Repeated stress and structural plasticity in the brain.* Ageing Res Rev. 2005 May;4(2):271-87.

Shankar SK. *Biology of aging brain.* Indian J Pathol Microbiol. 2010 Oct-Dec;53(4):595-604.

Zieliński K. *Jerzy Konorski on brain associations.* Acta Neurobiol Exp (Wars). 2006;66(1):75-84; discussion 85-90, 95-7.

AMYGDALA NEUROPLASTICITY

Hölzel BK, Carmody J, Vangel M, Congleton C, Yerramsetti SM, Gard T, Lazar SW. *Mindfulness practice leads to increases in regional brain gray matter density.* Psychiatry Res. 2011 Jan 30;191(1):36-43. Epub 2010 Nov 10.

Johnson RT, Breedlove SM, Jordan CL. *Astrocytes in the amygdala.* Vitam Horm. 2010;82:23-45.

Roozendaal B, McEwen BS, Chattarji S. *Stress, memory and the amygdala.* Nat Rev Neurosci. 2009 Jun;10(6):423-33.

DEEP BELLY BREATHING

Brown RP, Gerbarg PL. *Yoga breathing, meditation, and longevity.* Ann N Y Acad Sci. 2009 Aug;1172:54-62. Review

Martarelli D, Cocchioni M, Scuri S, Pompei P. *Diaphragmatic Breathing Reduces Exercise-induced Oxidative Stress.* Evid Based Complement Alternat Med. 2009 Oct 29.

MEDITATION

Carmody J, Baer RA. *Relationships between mindfulness practice and levels of mindfulness, medical and psychological symptoms and well-being in a mindfulness-based stress reduction program.* J Behav Med. 2008 Feb;31(1):23-33. Epub 2007 Sep 25.

Hölzel BK, Carmody J, Vangel M, Congleton C, Yerramsetti SM, Gard T, Lazar SW. *Mindfulness practice leads to increases in regional brain gray matter density.* Psychiatry Res. 2011 Jan 30;191(1):36-43. Epub 2010 Nov 10.

Hölzel BK, Ott U, Gard T, Hempel H, Weygandt M, Morgen K, Vaitl D. *Investigation of mindfulness meditation practitioners with voxel-based morphometry.* Soc Cogn Affect Neurosci. 2008 Mar;3(1):55-61. Epub 2007 Dec 3.

Schmidt S, Grossman P, Schwarzer B, Jena S, Naumann J, Walach H. *Treating fibromyalgia with mindfulness-based stress reduction: results from a 3-armed randomized controlled trial.* Pain. 2011 Feb;152(2):361-9. Epub 2010 Dec 13.

Thomley BS, Ray SH, Cha SS, Bauer BA. *Effects of a brief, comprehensive, yoga-based program on quality of life and biometric measures in an employee population: a pilot study.* Explore (NY). 2011 Jan-Feb;7(1):27-9.

POSITIVE PSYCHOLOGY

Adams O. *Life expectancy in Canada – an overview.* Health Rep. 1990;2(4):361-76.

Ballas D, Dorling D. *Measuring the impact of major life events upon happiness.* Int J Epidemiol. 2007 Dec;36(6):1244-52. Epub 2007 Sep 28.

Borgonovi F. *Doing well by doing good. The relationship between formal volunteering and self-reported health and happiness.* Soc Sci Med. 2008 Jun;66(11):2321-34. Epub 2008 Mar 5.

Chida Y, Steptoe A. *The association of anger and hostility with future coronary heart disease: a meta-analytic review of prospective evidence.* J Am Coll Cardiol. 2009 Mar 17;53(11):936-46.

Chida Y, Steptoe A. Psychobiology Group, Department of Epidemiology and Public Health, University College London, 1-19 Torrington Place, London, United Kingdom. y.chida@ucl.ac.uk *Positive psychological well-being and mortality: a quantitative review of prospective observational studies.* Psychosom Med. 2008 Sep;70(7):741-56. Epub 2008 Aug 25.

Costa PT Jr, McCrae RR. *Influence of extraversion and neuroticism on subjective well-being: happy and unhappy people.* J Pers Soc Psychol. 1980 Apr;38(4):668-78.

Csikszentmihalyi, Mihaly (1975). *Beyond Boredom and Anxiety: Experiencing Flow in Work and Play.* San Francisco: Jossey-Bass. ISBN 0-87589-261-2

Csikszentmihalyi, Mihaly (1998). *Finding Flow: The Psychology of Engagement With Everyday Life.* Basic Books. ISBN 0-465-02411-4

DeNeve KM, Cooper H. *The happy personality: a meta-analysis of 137 personality traits and subjective well-being.* Psychol Bull. 1998 Sep;124(2):197-229.

Diener E, Seligman ME. *Very happy people.* Psychol Sci. 2002 Jan;13(1):81-4.

Lykken DT. Department of Psychology, University of Minnesota, Minneapolis 55455, USA. *A more accurate estimate of heritability.* Twin Res Hum Genet. 2007 Feb;10(1):168-73.

Macht M, Dettmer D. *Everyday mood and emotions after eating a chocolate bar or an apple.* Appetite. 2006 May;46(3):332-6. Epub 2006 Mar 20.

Martin E P Seligman and Mihaly Csikszentmihalyi, guest editors. Satterfield JM. *Happiness, excellence, and optimal human functioning.* Review of a special issue of the American Psychologist (2000;55:5-183). West J Med. 2001 Jan;174(1):26-9.

Nutt D, Demyttenaere K, Janka Z, Aarre T, Bourin M, Canonico PL, Carrasco JL, Stahl S. *The other face of depression, reduced positive affect: the role of catecholamines in causation and cure.* J Psychopharmacol. 2007 Jul;21(5):461-71. Epub 2006 Oct 18.

Seligman ME. *How to see the glass half full.* Newsweek. 2002 Sep 16;140(12):48-9.

Seligman, Martin E.P.; Csikszentmihalyi, Mihaly (2000). *Positive Psychology: An Introduction.* American Psychologist 55 (1): 5–14.

Strobel M, Tumasjan A, Spörrle M. Munich University of Technology, Germany University of Applied Management Erding, Germany. *Be yourself, believe in yourself, and be happy: Self-efficacy as a mediator between personality factors and subjective well-being.* Scand J Psychol. 2011 Feb;52(1):43-8. doi: 10.1111/j.1467-9450.2010.00826.x.

CHAPTER 6

Human Hardware

SCN=Suprachiasmatic Nucleus

Hypothalam

Optic Nerve

Light in

Pituitary gland

Spinal C

Signal to Body

Panc

Heart

SCN

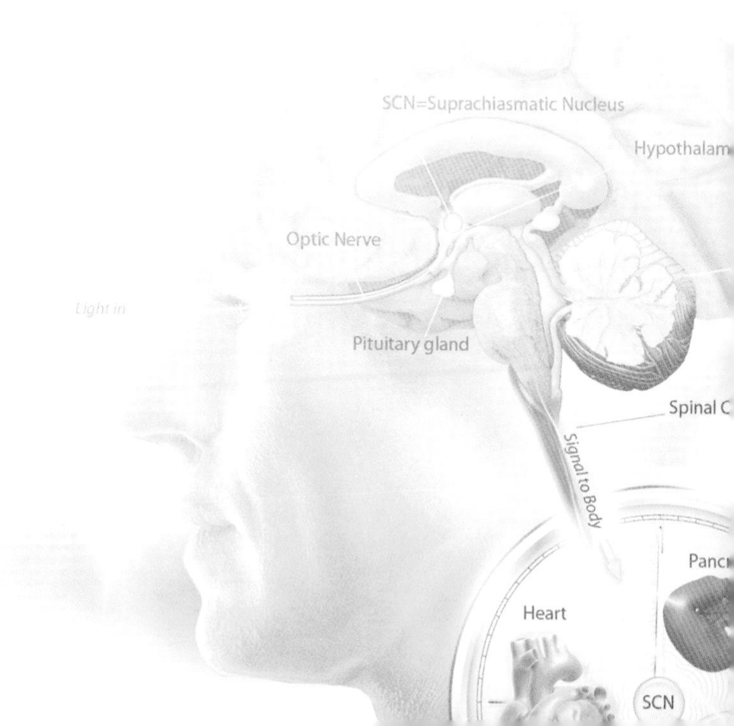

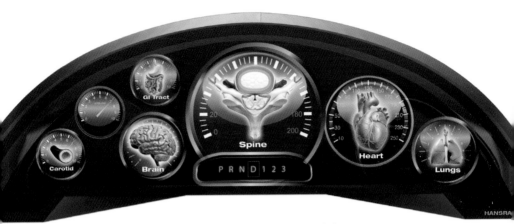

YOUR SPINAL HEALTH
IS THE KEY INDICATOR ON
THE DASHBOARD OF YOUR LIFE

THE SPINE IS A PRINCIPAL indicator of general health. Studies appear each day that confirm the negative impact poor spine health has on other parts of the body.

Spinal health is heavily influenced by one's inner world, outer world, and physical and emotional health. Everything from living a purposeful life, being in touch with personal goals, and understanding how the human brain and spine work to common everyday factors such as meditation, sleep, deep breathing, posture, outlook, drug and alcohol use, diet and exercise all influence spinal health.

Mastering spinal health will improve one's quality of life. Identify and work on the inner world, which is the human thought that runs the human body, and identify and work on your outer world. Happiness, sense of well being, and personal health will improve with a focus on both these worlds.

CAROTID ARTERY
INTIMAL MEDIA THICKNESS

CAROTID ATHEROSCLEROSIS or INTIMA-MEDIA THICK-NESS (IMT): IMT is the breadth of the innermost layer of the carotid artery. Since they have similar risk factors, the carotid arteries provide a "window" to the condition of the coronary arteries and subsequent risk for stroke and heart disease. Further studies have identified relationships with sciatica (leg pain due to nerve dysfunction), lumbar spine bone mass in postmenopausal women, and osteoporosis. Carotid artery thickening offers a glimpse of the degree of coronary artery thickening (atherosclerosis) in an individual. IMT is an independent predictor of future cardiovascular problems such as heart attacks, cardiac death and stroke.

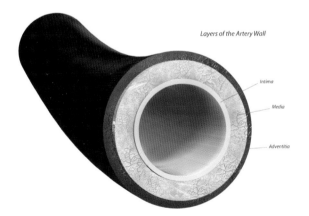

Layers of the Artery Wall

Intima

Media

Adventitia

Recent studies have shown that sciatica (leg pain due to nerve dysfunction) could be a manifestation of IMT or that both conditions might share common risk factors. Literature from other studies have reported IMT being directly related to the amount of blood that flows within a vertebral body. The thicker the intima-media, the less blood delivered to the artery of the vertebra.

Intima-media thickness might be associated with the loss of lumbar spine bone mass in postmenopausal women. This suggests that postmenopausal women with osteoporosis could have a more aggressive IMT than those with normal bone mass.

IMT is driven by hypertension and diabetes and new studies are underway to assess its role in brain function, especially concerning the prediction of Alzheimer's. Lifestyle options can significantly improve hypertension and diabetes, resulting in the slowed thickening of the carotid artery intima-media.

AVOID BENDING, LIFTING, TWISTING, AND REACHING WHEN YOU ARE IN PAIN

When a herniated disc is compressing a nerve and the nerve is enflamed it makes sense to avoid bending, lifting, twisting and reaching as much as possible. These actions diminish the mobility of the compressed nerve. Nerve mobility treatments are started when the inflammation is reduced.

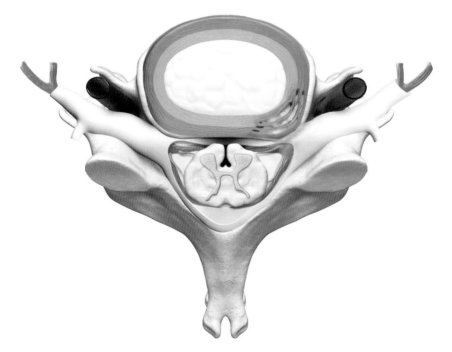

POSTURE

Posture describes the attitude or position of the body in a particular space. Posture is critical to the rehabilitation of the cervical spine and living a pain-free life.

Neutral spine is the proper alignment of the body between postural extremes in its most balanced position. Keep in mind that the spine is not a straight line; it has curves in the cervical (neck), thoracic (mid-back), and lumbar(lower back) regions. Neutral spine serves to reduce the stress that the facet joints, spinal cord, nerve roots, vertebra and muscles experience. It is also the most efficient position.

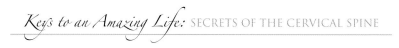

GOOD POSTURE

Good posture may be defined as ears being placed above the shoulders, and the "angel wings" or the scapula retracted.

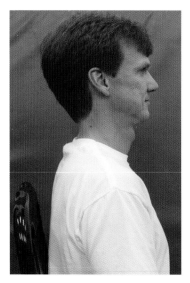

Head Over Shoulder

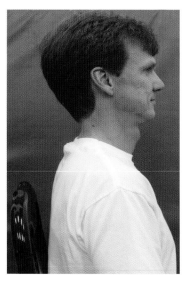

Cervical Lordosis

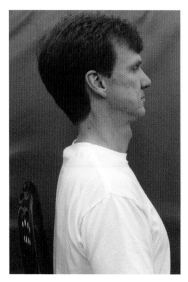

Squared Shoulder

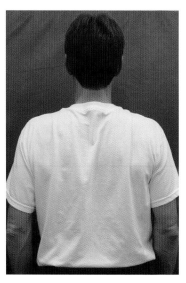

Retracted Scapula

BAD POSTURE

Bad posture may be defined as the droop of the head forward or the droop of the shoulders forward.

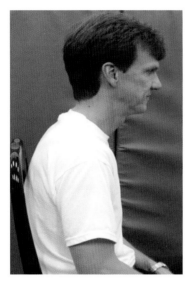

Head Tilted Forward

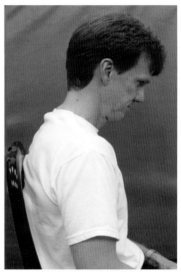

Cervical Kyphosis

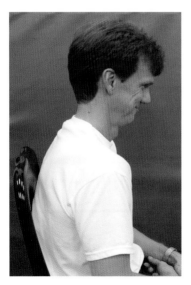

Rounded Shoulder

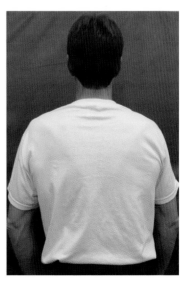

Protracted Scapula

REACHING

Reaching is difficult with a cervical nerve or spinal cord compression, especially neuroforaminal or central stenosis. Repetitive reaching motions cause nerves to be mobilized through tight canals which leads to pain and discomfort. After decades of painting, Leon G. found that it was easier on his nerves if he raised himself closer to his work with a ladder instead of reaching to paint. Being closer to the job adjusts his neck from extension (tighter canal) to flexion (allowing more space for nerve roots). The act of reaching tends to make tight nerves symptomatic. By eliminating extensive reaching, Leon was able to prolong his career another ten years.

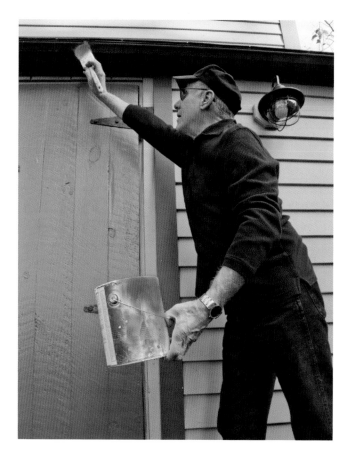

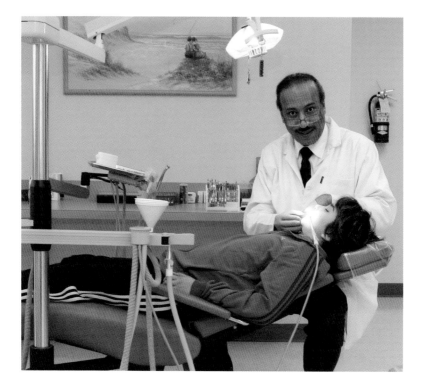

DENTISTS

Dentists are at an increased risk of experiencing excessive wear of the neck. Different studies have reported that as few as 26% and as many as 90% of dentists experience neck or back pain. An even greater percentage of hygienists have been found to encounter these problems. Some of these findings have been documented as early as dental school. Dental careers have been cut short due to spine problems while others never began. Static awkward posture (same posture that is held throughout the exertion), particularly with isometric contractions of the trapezius (large, superficial muscle that spans the neck, shoulders and back), has been identified as a specific risk factor. Ergonomically improved chairs appear to have some positive impact and I believe they will help reduce the stress experienced by the neck and upper extremities. However, studies have not yet confirmed these results.

NURSES

Nurses are at a high risk of wearing out their necks and backs. This profession involves a lot of bending, lifting, twisting and reaching. As obesity is on the rise, nurses are required to lift and move increasingly heavier patients. Many years of long hours of nursing might lead to deconditioning and wear and tear of the spine. Studies suggest that approximately 50% of nurses develop significant neck and back pain.

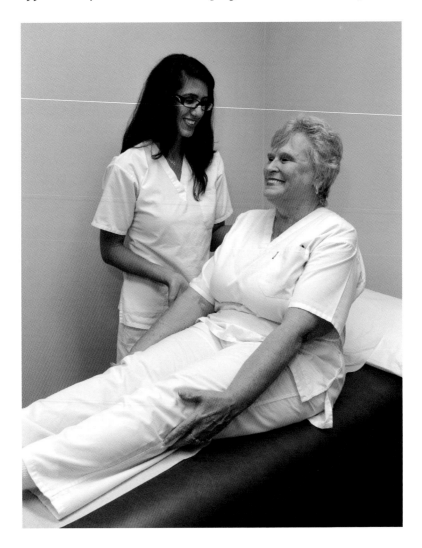

HAIRSTYLISTS

Hairstylists wear out their necks by using scissors, combs, hairdryers, etc. in one position, repetitively, for extended periods. A typical stylist could make up to an average of 30 scissor cuts per minute for 5 hours a day, 5 days a week, 50 weeks per year. That would be an estimated 2,250,000 cuts per year with the neck and arms in static positions.

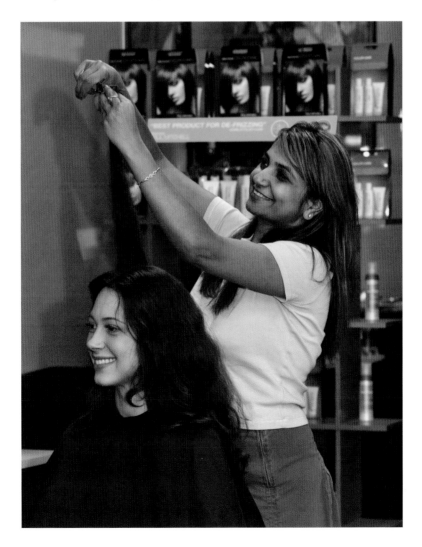

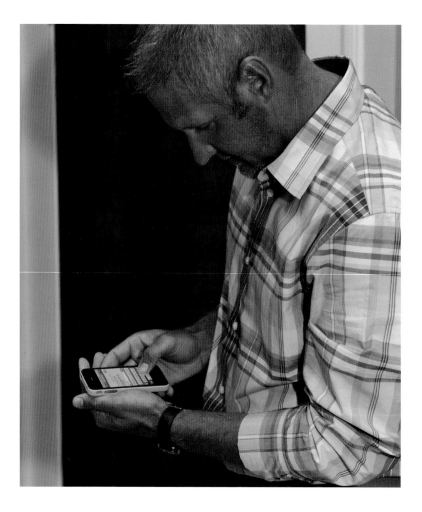

TEXTING

Text Neck refers to the strain that occurs in the muscles of the neck and shoulders from constantly looking down to send or receive text messages. Texters should text with the neck in the neutral position. Texting from a neutral spine position with attention to cervical stabilization will prevent pain and injury that could become permanent with time.

Blackberry Neck is defined by lingo as the distinctive pattern of unsightly creases and wrinkles caused by spending hours with a bent neck, looking down at one's smartphone.

LABORERS

Carpenters, masons, carpet and tile installers, construction workers, building inspectors, equipment operators, drywall and ceiling specialists electricians, elevator installers, glaziers, material deconstruction, painters, plumbers, roofers, sheet metal workers, iron workers and wreckers are but just a few of our types of workers in the physical labor field.

Bending, twisting, heavy lifting, and reaching for a lifetime can take its toll on the human body. Most tradespeople need help with their neck and back from time to time. A smaller percentage proceed to elect surgery. Careers are shortened with cumulative and progressive back and neck injuries.

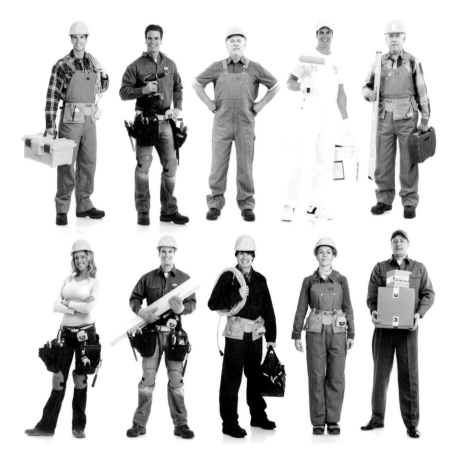

WELDERS

In my practice, I have met with welders that are stuck in the same static awkward posture hours a day for years. They look up and down and side to side while wearing heavy masks. Typically, we try to develop strategies to protect and strengthen their bodies, enhance their rest and prolong their career.

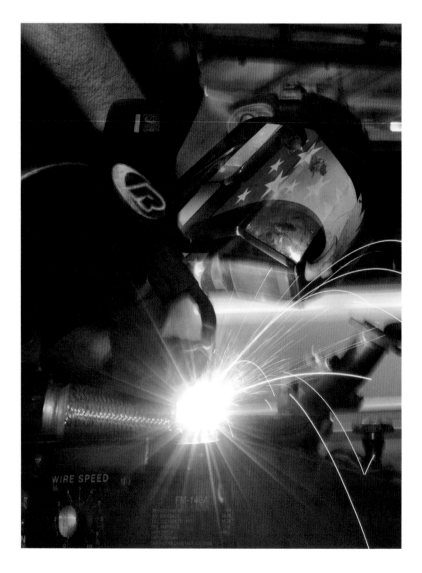

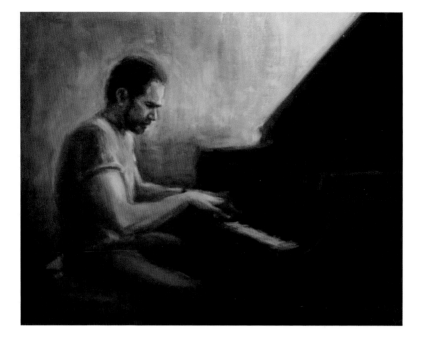

PIANISTS

Famous New York Pianist Robert Mosci has a work history of 25 years full time piano playing. His work amounts to playing piano 5 times a week, 4 hours a night, 40 minutes on, 20 minutes off and therefore approximately 3 hours per night. We calculated that he has played professionally approximately 18,750 hours of piano and definitely more with practice. He complained of neck pain and stiffness as well as right wrist and index finger pain when playing.

His MRI scan of the cervical spine was essentially normal, while his EMG showed a mild left C7 radiculopathy as well as a mild right-sided carpal tunnel syndrome.

To help Robert Mosci with his inner world, we recommended being careful with positive and negative thinking, diminishing stresses about his life and to employ the strategies of silence, solitude and stillness.

Recommended lifestyle changes include employing good posture, using long hot showers, developing a sleeping sanctuary, taking time off during the day for a mid-day nap, and taking a day off per week for rest and relaxation.

In his physical, outer world, he was recommended to employ good posture, do whole body stretches including hamstring stretches, yoga with emphasis on upward dog and downward dog and facet mobilization techniques. Vitamin B-Complex and Omega-3 supplementation were recommended.

This case study presents a unique opportunity to display strategies recommended to prolong and augment a very important career.

Air

A DEEP BREATH OF CLEAN FRESH AIR
IS AS SOOTHING TO THE BODY AS
A LARGE GLASS OF COOL WATER
ON A HOT SUMMER DAY.

DEEP BELLY BREATHING

DEEP BREATHING serves to improve the motion of the spinal segments, spinal cord and nerve roots, and it increases the cerebrospinal fluid motion and distribution.

Deep breathing might also decrease the swelling of the deranged joint and possibly the nerve root.

Deep breathing leads to improve disc hydration and osmotic motion, which helps healing factors such as oxygen and nutrition travel to the disk and joint in greater quantities.

Breathing techniques may be found many places online. The Art of Living Foundation may be a good source to begin with (www.artofliving.org).

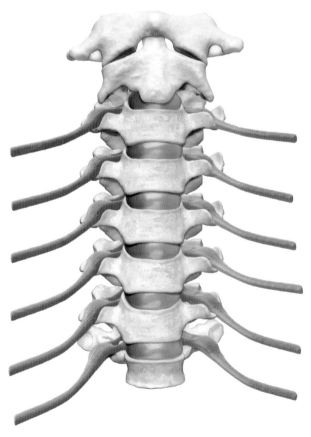

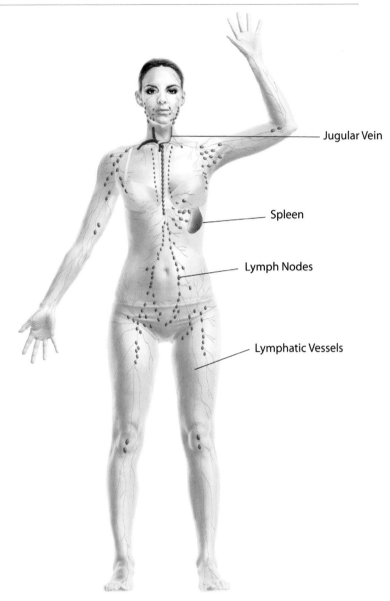

Jugular Vein

Spleen

Lymph Nodes

Lymphatic Vessels

Deep breathing also improves and increases lymphatic flow which contributes in the aid of the inflammatory response. The lymphatic system is part of the immune system that comprises a network of conduits called lymphatic vessels that transport immune cells to and from the lymph nodes. The lymphatic system is one that is separate from that of the arteries and veins.

WORKPLACE COMFORT

ARCHITECTS ARE KNOWN to be among the most common sufferers of neck pain. This profession requires many hours of sitting in the same position creating initial building designs on computers. Careers may be lengthened and enhanced by paying attention to the factors mentioned in this book.

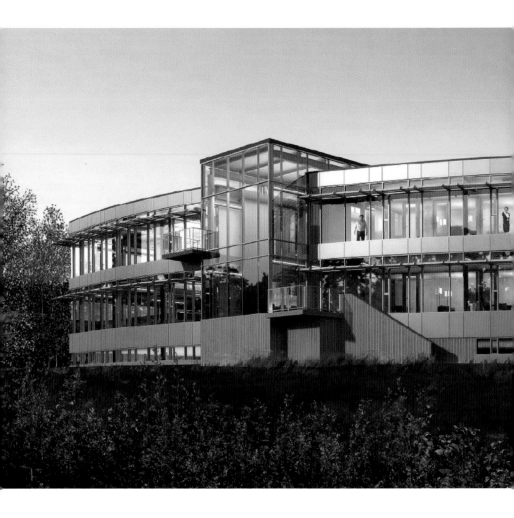

World class architects are designing better buildings. Workspaces are being created to provide daylight without glare, sunlight, fresh air, normal pressure air delivery as opposed to high pressure forced air, and flexible workspaces with personalized air supply.

Toronto based master architect Dermot Sweeny (www.andco.com) has designed some 6,000,000 square feet of high performance human comfort workspaces. Future studies might find that special attention to building design results in less pain and suffering, and improved happiness and performance in the workplace.

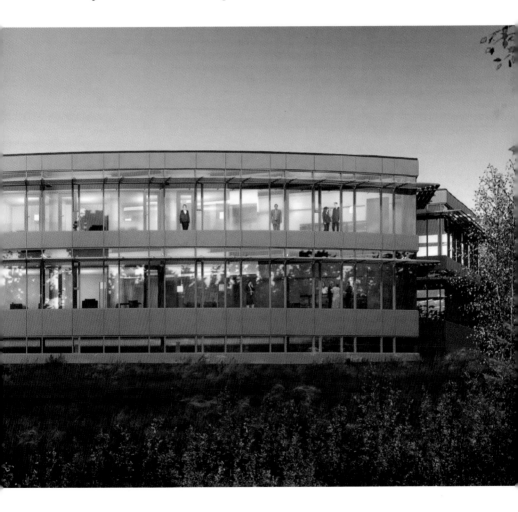

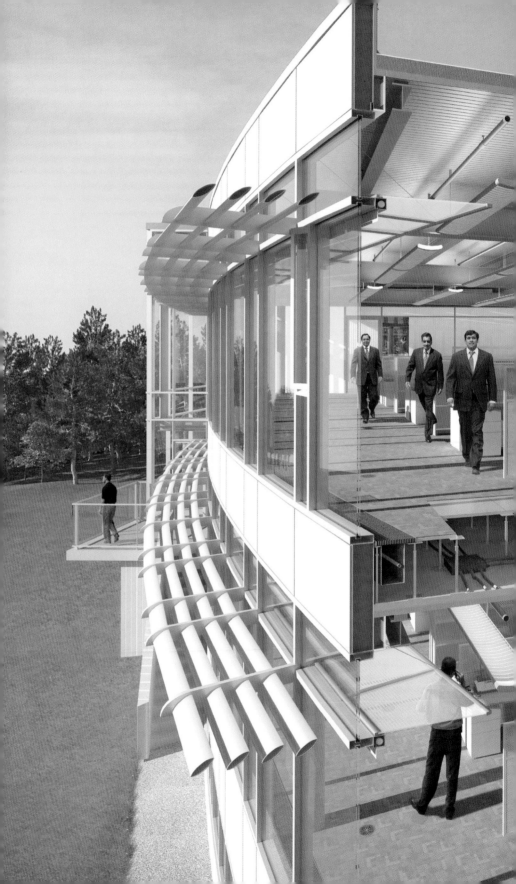

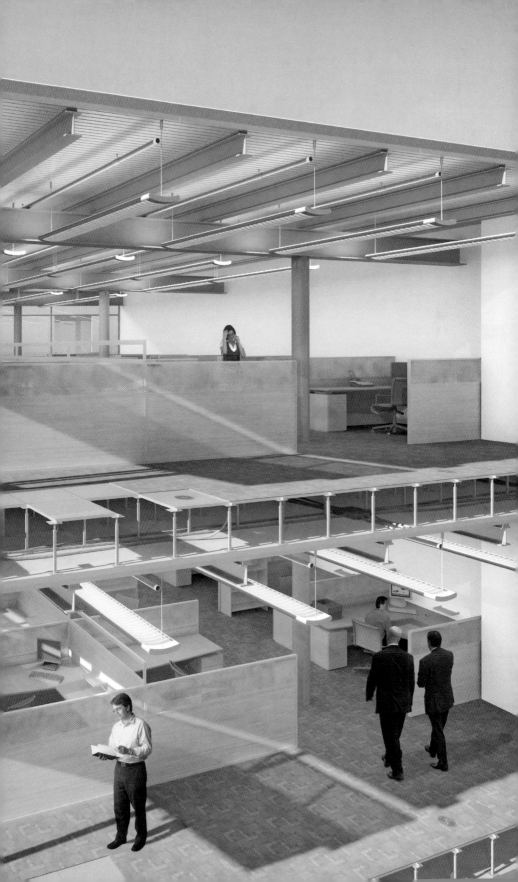

WATER

G ENERAL RECOMMENDATIONS for hydration are 8 eight-ounce glasses of water per day. Current recommendations for hydration are to drink between ½ an ounce to 1 ounce of water daily for each pound of body weight. For example, if you weigh 170 pounds then you should consume 85 to 170 ounces of water a day. Associated factors of hot or cold weather, dry climate, high altitude, alcohol use, exercise, pregnancy, and sickness lead to increase need for water.

SOURCES

Water is natural and hydrates better than any other liquid.

Sports Drinks are full of electrolytes (substances that become ions in solution and acquire the capacity to conduct electricity)and are a tastier option than water but could lead to increased consumption. These drinks are laden with sugars and hidden calories.

Juice has vitamins, minerals, and electrolytes but is high in sugar. Sugars reduce water absorption, making juice a poor hydration option.

Soda tastes great; however, it is a poor thirst quencher. The presence of caffeine and sugar will provide a short-term energy boost but, ultimately, will slow the absorption of water.

Coffee and Tea are diuretics which work to expel water from the body. Added milk or sugar will further reduce water absorption.

Alcohol dehydrates the body, removes necessary electrolytes and interrupts the Krebs Cycle (a series of chemical enzymatic reactions that catalyzes the aerobic metabolism of fuel molecules to carbon dioxide and water, generating energy from the production of ATP).

Studies do suggest that appropriate hydration significantly decreases the risk for:

+ colon cancer
+ breast cancer
+ bladder cancer

LONG HOT SHOWERS
(OR COLD SHOWERS IN HOT COUNTRIES)

A LONG, HOT SHOWER acts as a stress reducer. Cleansing not only removes dirt and debris from the body, but it removes emotional burden as well. Wash with the intent to remove both physical and mental grime. Muscles start to relax and heal, enhancing a day's work or a night's sleep. In times of stress and pain, I recommend showering two times per day. In the deep winter, many of my clients report that they "empty the hot water tank."

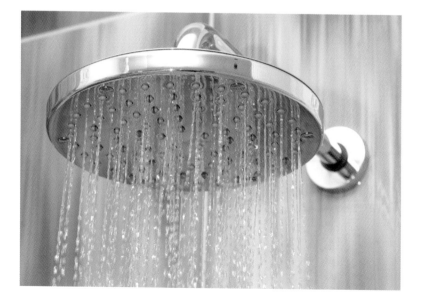

PLANNING

*"I dream my painting
and I paint my dream."*

VINCENT VAN GOGH

PLAN YOUR HOURS, days, and weeks. The more planned your life is, the less stress there is to be encountered. Many of my clients find day planning helpful in protecting their spine. Begin your morning with a long, hot shower for cleansing and warming of the spinal joints and muscles. Reflection and meditation lead to a thoughtful day. Think through your activities and meetings. Schedule private moments, especially a midday nap whenever possible. End your day with another long, hot shower.

BED REST

COUNTERINTUITIVE but necessary, 1-2 days of bed rest may be considered for acute pain. Studies have shown that prolonged bed rest might be detrimental in the overall recovery from back pain, including sciatica.

Early to bed and early to rise makes a man healthy, wealthy and wise.

Benjamin Franklin

WAKE UP TIME

O UR PARENTS and ancestors advised us to wake up early, a recommendation that science supports. Since the body is hormonally and metabolically boosted early in the morning, it can do more and think better. Performance is also enhanced during these early hours since "the rest of the world is sleeping."

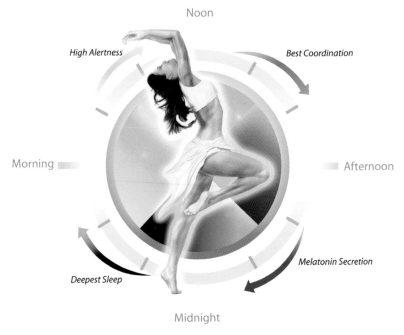

Master Clock

The circadian rhythm describes the endogenously driven 24-hour cycle in biochemical, physiological and behavioral processes. In other words, this means our waking and sleeping cycles. The word "circadian" comes from the phrase "circa diem," which translates to about a day or twenty-four hours.

The body has a master clock consisting of approximately 20,000 nerve cells in the hypothalamus portion of the brain that coordinates

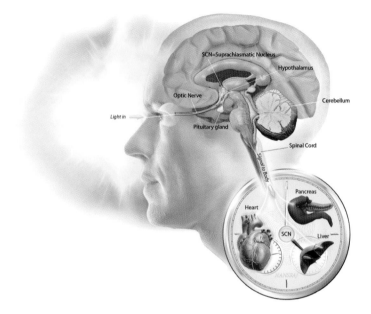

signals called the suprachiasmatic nucleus (SCN). The retinas, multi-layered sensory tissue that line the back of the eye, contain photosensitive cells that send light information to the SCN. The SCN then relays a message to the pineal gland, a small pinecone-shaped organ located on the midline and attached to the posterior end of the roof of the third ventricle of the brain. The pineal gland secretes melatonin, a structurally simple hormone that communicates information about environmental lighting to various parts of the body.

The elementary pattern is that serum concentrations of melatonin begin to increase once the sun sets and serum concentrations decrease to lower serum levels during the day. Melatonin has important effects on sleep-wake cycles, reproduction, and functions presenting circadian rhythm.

The SCN prepares the body for the upcoming day with an anticipatory rise in heart rate, glucose, and cortisol. Cortisol, a steroid hormone, or glucocorticoid, produced by the adrenal gland, reaches its lowest level between midnight and 4 am, or 3 to 5 hours after the onset of sleep. Peak levels occur in the early morning around 8 am, the same time melatonin levels decrease.

SLEEP

SLEEP STUDIES SUGGEST that insufficient sleep is associated with increased neck and back problems; impaired driving performance and thinking function; mood related problems in children, adolescents, and adults; impaired judgment in medical residents; depression; and earlier death due to cardiac-related problems. Insufficient sleep might lead to obstructed sleep apnea. Left untreated it could lead to a transient ischemic attack (TIA), a "mini stroke" or "warning stroke," and, subsequently, stroke.

Recent studies concluded that consistently sleeping too long (9 or more hours per night) is as detrimental to one's health as sleeping too little (6 hours or less per night) and could, ultimately, contribute to early death.

Studies also suggest that adequate sleep is associated with making more healthful food choices. Eating right plays a significant role in the

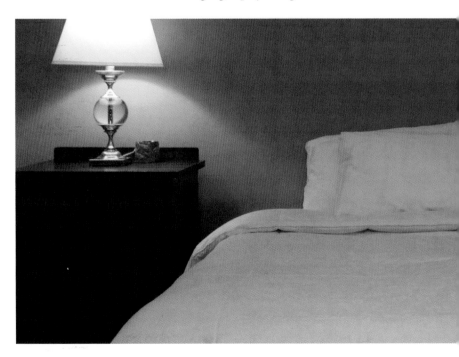

prevention of obesity, especially in children, and is key player in the fight against heart disease.

Sleep is an extremely important factor in the spinal derivative. Worldwide, people do not sleep enough or are not able to achieve a deep, restful and restorative sleep. Create a sanctuary for sleep and carefully choose the correct mattress and pillow for comfort. Use drapes or blinds to eliminate all outdoor light; close all closets leading to, or near, the bedroom to prevent sleeping in a bath of dry cleaning chemicals; provide fresh, cool sleeping temperature air; and avoid the use of electronics, such as a television and radio, and power off cellphones.

I remember consulting a Pepsi executive who was not sleeping well due to her husband's blackberry email and text notifications that sounded throughout the night. Also, electronics might cause electromagnetic interference, though the effects on human beings is not yet clear.

Colors of the bedroom, linens and drapes should be calming and

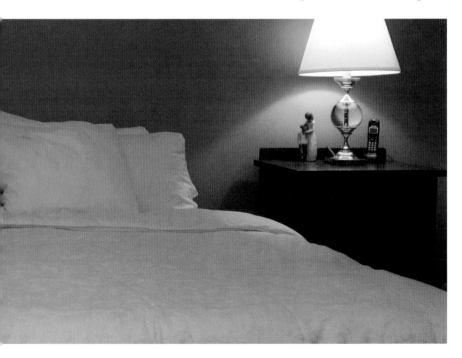

pleasing. Mattresses are a personal choice. Some clients sleep well on firm surfaces, while others sleep better on soft surfaces. Main body parts are supported by a firm mattress, however the joint areas are better padded by a softer layer. Experiment with the softness, material content and functionality of different pillows. Some pillows are made to recess at pressure points.

I love to sleep on my side with two pillows under my head to keep my neck straight. Try using a firm base pillow and a softer top pillow. Also, use pillows liberally between arms and legs or, perhaps, under the back.

HOURS OF SLEEP

The correct amount of sleep is the amount that provides a refreshed feeling. For me, 7 to 8 hours per night seems to be the correct number, however, operating a busy medical practice sometimes only allows me to get 4 or 5 hours. When this happens on occasion for a few days, I usually allow myself a 12-hour night of sleep or a few naps in the day when my schedule returns to normal.

Mumbai-based architect Ninad Tipnis specializes in world class LEED (Leadership in Energy & Environmental Design) certification of interior fit-outs. Ninad lives a purpose-driven life. He wakes at 4:30, performs a "holy hour" of day and life planning, followed by an hour of exercise. Ninad sets an alarm to remind himself when it's time to eat due to his non-stop schedule. He is out like a light every night at 9.

If you have created a good sleeping environment; taken a long, hot shower; engaged in deep breathing; tried being purposeful and intent about sleeping, and you are still unable to do so, consider a sleeping aid. Try meditation or using white noise (a signal or process that contains equal power within a fixed bandwidth at any center frequency). Some examples of white noise are a waterfall, rain shower, fan, or wind blowing through the trees. The sounds are used to calm a busy mind or distract the mind from neural stimulators heard inside or outside the home. White noise machines can be purchased, as well as white noise apps for smartphones. Further yet, brainwave entrainment engineer Morry Zelcovitch has developed a sequence of tones that mechanically augments sleep. For those suffering from long periods of insomnia, I recommend cranial osteopathy. This hands-on treatment induces a deep sleep that would be deeply restful and may break the stressful or painful cycle.

Not all sleep medications are necessarily your friend. Melatonin is a naturally occurring hormone found in humans that might allow the entrainment of the circadian rhythm and enhance sleep. Diphenhydramine, commonly known as the brand name Benadryl®, contains one of several antihistamines used for the treatment of seasonal allergies. This drug is one of the most common used medications to enhance sleep. However, drugs like Benadryl®, Nyquil®, Excedrin PM®, and alcohol will cause drowsiness but will also prevent the brain from entering the REM (rapid eye movement) stage of sleep. This often leaves a person feeling tired the next day. Although a continued topic of debate, some studies have suggested that only experiencing non-REM stages of sleep for long periods might lead to memory impairment.

For profound sleep disorders, a physician might recommend prescription strength psychotropic sleep medications such as benzodiazepine. Psychotropics could be related to drug dependence, withdrawal syndrome, inadequate quality of sleep, and the risk of birth defects in women of child-bearing age.

NAP

THE BRAIN NEEDS a nap, which is a short period of sleep, in the afternoon approximately between 2 to 4 pm. Napping is beneficial in restoring alertness, boosting mood, improving productivity and prolonging life. Naps can be enhanced with warmth, fresh air, soft music or, my favorite, meditation.

I might do a guided imagery meditation piece for 15 minutes and a nap for an additional 15 minutes. Otherwise, I fall asleep with a brainwave entrainment audio piece through a headset or, better yet, a full stereo system to feel the sound waves.

NERVE MOBILITY

THE LONGER I have my medical practice the more I appreciate the concept of nerve mobility. The nerves extending from the canals are noted to be mobile with every breath we take. While in surgery, the anesthesiologist will sometimes perform a valsalva maneuver, which is a very deep artificial breathing. That is when the nerves are at their most mobile state.

Herniated discs could impinge and inflame spinal nerves. The combination of diminished nerve mobility and inflammation leads to a very painful result. In revision surgery we do come across cases of nerves being stuck by a scar and losing their mobility. When the nerve is freed, typically, the patient is better. Therefore, nerve mobility is important to the well-being of the spine. Deep belly breathing, nerve mobilization techniques and yoga are among the best techniques to enhance nerve mobility.

FACET MOBILITY

At every level of the spine there are joints called the facet joints that are, in my opinion, the cornerstone of the spine.

Facets, which provide the spine its flexibility, are truly joints with a fibrous capsule and synovial fluid. These joints are similar to those found in the knee or hip.

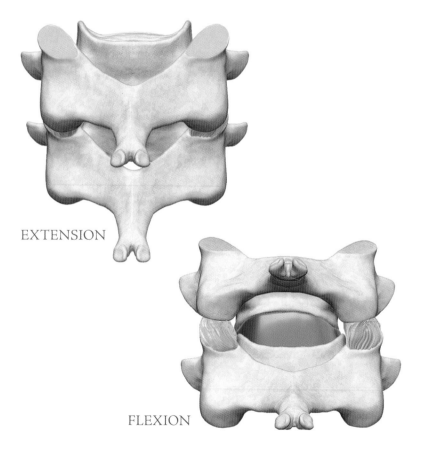

EXTENSION

FLEXION

The top left figure shows the posterior view of the facet joint in an extension position, while the bottom right figure shows the facet joint in a flexion position from the posterior view.

The facet joints form the posterior wall of the access way for the nerve to leave the spine. It is important to keep these joints mobile and supple to prevent nerve and facet joint dysfunction. Chiropractors and osteopaths specialize in techniques to keep the joints limber. Yoga, Pilates, and cervical and lumbar stabilization all serve to provide range of motion and strengthening especially for the spine's facet joints. Dietary supplements glucosamine and chondroitin sulfate could allow for reduced doses of non-steroidal anti-inflammatory agents in cases of arthritis of the facet joints.

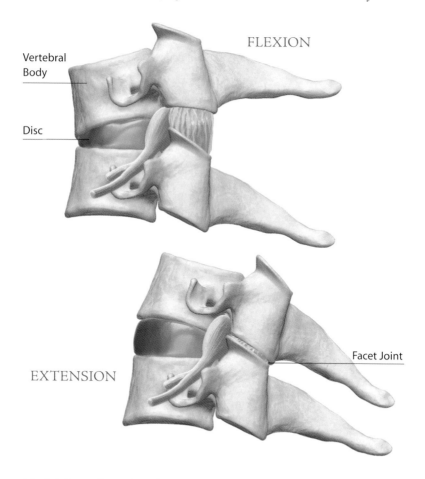

FLEXION

Vertebral Body

Disc

Facet Joint

EXTENSION

The left figure shows the side view of the facet joint in a flexion position, while the right figure shows the facet joint in an extension position from the side view.

HUMAN SEXUALITY
AND THE SPINE

HUMAN SEXUALITY is the accumulation of good results of great lifestyle implementations, and of managing the inner and outer worlds. The physical act of copulation is a great manifestation of upward and downward dog yoga poses. The upward and downward dog positions employ hyperflexion and hyperextension of the spinal column, respectively. The mobility of the facet joint is quite important in implementing sexual techniques.

Safe techniques, when in pain, include a stabilized spine and the elimination of bending and twisting. So, the person suffering from a spinal injury may lie on the ground while their partner is on top. Otherwise, the suffering person may lie on a table with their partner holding the suffering person's legs for support.

The missionary position is the most difficult with back pain and, probably, should be avoided. Props such as a lumbar support or a pillow under the back could help.

The desire of copulation represents physical health producing base hormones such as the libido driving testosterone and estrogen. The act of copulation leads to increased dopamine and serotonin secretion in the brain, leading to the physical experience of feeling good and happy. Oxytocin secretion leads to a bonding feeling.

BIBLIOGRAPHY

CAROTID ARTERY INTIMAL MEDIA THICKNESS

Celiloglu M, Aydin Y, Balci P, Kolamaz T. *The effect of alendronate sodium on carotid artery intima-media thickness and lipid profile in women with postmenopausal osteoporosis.* Menopause. 2009 Jul-Aug;16(4):689-93.

Chen WT, Ting-Fang Shih T, Hu CJ, Chen RC, Tu HY. *Relationship between vertebral bone marrow blood perfusion and common carotid intima-media thickness in aging adults.* J Magn Reson Imaging. 2004 Nov;20(5):811-6.

Hmamouchi I, Allali F, Khazzani H, Bennani L, El Mansouri L, Ichchou L, Cherkaoui M, Abouqal R, Hajjaj-Hassouni N. *Low bone mineral density is related to atherosclerosis in postmenopausal Moroccan women.* BMC Public Health. 2009 Oct 14;9:388.

Saleh C. *Carotid artery intima media thickness: a predictor of cognitive impairment?* Front Biosci (Elite Ed). 2010 Jun 1;2:980-90.

Shiri R, Viikari-Juntura E, Leino-Arjas P, Vehmas T, Varonen H, Moilanen L, Karppinen J, Heliövaara M. *The association between carotid intima-media thickness and sciatica.* Semin Arthritis Rheum. 2007 Dec;37(3):174-81. Epub 2007 May 15.

Tamaki J, Iki M, Hirano Y, Sato Y, Kajita E, Kagamimori S, Kagawa Y and Yoneshima H. *Low bone mass is associated with carotid atherosclerosis in postmenopausal women: The Japanese Population-based Osteoporosis (JPOS) Cohort Study.* Osteoporosis International, Volume 20, Number 1, 53-60, DOI: 10.1007/s00198-008-0633-z

DENTISTS

Abiodun-Solanke IM, Agbaje JO, Ajayi DM, Arotiba JT. *Prevalence of neck and back pain among dentists and dental auxiliaries in South-western Nigeria.* Afr J Med Med Sci. 2010 Jun;39(2):137-42.

Al Wazzan KA, Almas K, Al Shethri SE, Al-Qahtani MQ. *Back & neck problems among dentists and dental auxiliaries.* J Contemp Dent Pract. 2001 Aug 15;2(3):17-30.

Diaz-Caballero AJ, Gómez-Palencia IP, Díaz-Cárdenas S. *Ergonomic factors that cause the presence of pain muscle in students of dentistry.* Med Oral Patol Oral Cir Bucal. 2010 Nov 1;15(6):e906-11.

Harutunian K, Gargallo-Albiol J, Figueiredo R, Gay-Escoda C. *Ergonomics and musculoskeletal pain among postgraduate students and faculty members of the School of Dentistry of the University of Barcelona (Spain). A cross-sectional study.* Med Oral Patol Oral Cir Bucal. 2010 Aug 15. [Epub ahead of print]

Lalumandier JA, McPhee SD, Parrott CB, Vendemia M. *Musculoskeletal pain: prevalence, prevention, and differences among dental office personnel.* Gen Dent. 2001 Mar-Apr;49(2):160-6.

Morse T, Bruneau H, Dussetschleger J. *Musculoskeletal disorders of the neck and shoulder in the dental professions.* Work. 2010;35(4):419-29.

NURSES

Charney W. *The need to legislate the health-care industry in the state of Washington to protect health-care workers from back injury.* J Long Term Eff Med Implants. 2005;15(5):567-72.

Hudson MA. *Texas passes first law for safe patient handling in America: landmark legislation protects health-care workers and patients from injury related to manual patient lifting.* J Long Term Eff Med Implants. 2005;15(5):559-66.

Silverstein B, Viikari-Juntura E, Kalat J. *Use of a prevention index to identify industries at high risk for work-related musculoskeletal disorders of the neck, back, and upper extremity in Washington state, 1990-1998.* Am J Ind Med. 2002 Mar;41(3):149-69.

Sveinsdóttir H, Biering P, Ramel A. *Occupational stress, job satisfaction, and working environment among Icelandic nurses: a cross-sectional questionnaire survey.* Int J Nurs Stud. 2006 Sep;43(7):875-89. Epub 2005 Dec 19.

Tinubu BM, Mbada CE, Oyeyemi AL, Fabunmi AA. *Work-related musculoskeletal disorders among nurses in Ibadan, South-west Nigeria: a cross-sectional survey.* BMC Musculoskelet Disord. 2010 Jan 20;11:12.

Trinkoff AM, Le R, Geiger-Brown J, Lipscomb J, Lang G. *Longitudinal relationship of work hours, mandatory overtime, and on-call to musculoskeletal problems in nurses.* Am J Ind Med. 2006 Nov;49(11):964-71.

van Soest EM, Fritschi L. *Occupational health risks in veterinary nursing: an exploratory study.* Aust Vet J. 2004 Jun;82(6):346-50.

BED REST

Verbunt JA, Sieben J, Vlaeyen JW, Portegijs P, André Knottnerus J. *A new episode of low back pain: who relies on bed rest?* Eur J Pain. 2008 May;12(4):508-16. Epub 2007 Sep 17.

WATER

Altieri A, La Vecchia C, Negri E. *Fluid intake and risk of bladder and other cancers.* Eur J Clin Nutr. 2003 Dec;57 Suppl 2:S59-68.

Altieri A, La Vecchia C, Negri E. *Fluid intake and risk of bladder and other cancers.* Eur J Clin Nutr. 2003 Dec;57 Suppl 2:S59-68.

Cowbrough K, Lloyd H. *A measurement and comparison of the fluid intake in people with and without back pain.* J Hum Nutr Diet. 2003 Dec;16(6):403-9.

Michaud DS, Spiegelman D, Clinton SK, Rimm EB, Curhan GC, Willett WC, Giovannucci EL. *Fluid intake and the risk of bladder cancer in men.* N Engl J Med. 1999 May 6;340(18):1390-7.

Michaud DS, Spiegelman D, Clinton SK, Rimm EB, Curhan GC, Willett WC, Giovannucci EL. *Fluid intake and the risk of bladder cancer in men.*N Engl J Med. 1999 May 6;340(18):1390-7.

WAKE UP TIME

Gangwisch JE. *Epidemiological evidence for the links between sleep, circadian rhythms and metabolism.* Obes Rev. 2009 Nov;10 Suppl 2:37-45.

Posener JA, Schildkraut JJ, Samson JA, Schatzberg AF. *Diurnal variation of plasma cortisol and homovanillic acid in healthy subjects.* Psychoneuroendocrinology. 1996 Jan;21(1):33-8.

Weitzman ED et al. *Twenty-four-hour Patterns of the Episodic Secretion of Cortisol in Normal Subjects.* Journal of Clinical Endocrinology and Metabolism, vol. 33, pp. 13–22, 1971

SLEEP

Cappuccio FP, D'Elia L, Strazzullo P, Miller MA. *Sleep duration and all-cause mortality: a systematic review and meta-analysis of prospective studies.* Sleep. 2010 May 1;33(5):585-92.

Cappuccio FP, Taggart FM, Kandala NB, Currie A, Peile E, Stranges S, Miller MA. *Meta-analysis of short sleep duration and obesity in children and adults.* Sleep. 2008 May 1;31(5):619-26.

Kopasz M, Loessl B, Hornyak M, Riemann D, Nissen C, Piosczyk H, Voderholzer U. *Sleep and memory in healthy children and adolescents – a critical review.* Sleep Med Rev. 2010 Jun;14(3):167-77. Epub 2010 Jan 25.

Metlaine A, Leger D, Choudat D. *Socioeconomic impact of insomnia in working populations.* Ind Health. 2005 Jan;43(1):11-9.

Olds T, Blunden S, Petkov J, Forchino F. *The relationships between sex, age, geography and time in bed in adolescents: a meta-analysis of data from 23 countries.* Sleep Med Rev. 2010 Dec;14(6):371-8. Epub 2010 Mar 6.

NAP

http://health.msn.com/health-topics/articlepage.aspx?cp-documentid=100233156&GT1=31036

"NASA Nap" 2005-06-03. 2007-08-24.

Anthony, Camile and William. *The Art of Napping at Work.* Larson Publication, 1999.

Mednick, Sara C.; Mark Ehrman (December 2006). *Take a Nap!* (First printing ed.). New York, NY, USA: Workman Publishing. pp. 133.

The National Institute of Mental Health Power Nap Study. 2002-07-01. Retrieved 2002-07-01.

NERVE MOBILITY

Gilbert KK, Brismée JM, Collins DL, James CR, Shah RV, Sawyer SF, Sizer PS Jr. *2006 Young Investigator Award Winner: lumbosacral nerve root displacement and strain: part 1. A novel measurement technique during straight leg raise in unembalmed cadavers.* Spine (Phila Pa 1976). 2007 Jun 15;32(14):1513-20.

CHAPTER 7

Social Choices

TOBACCO
ALCOHOL
DRUG USE

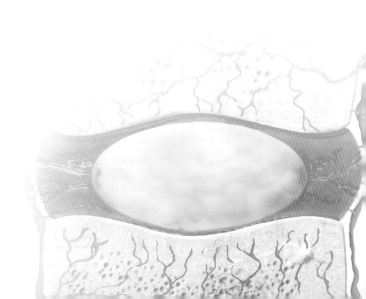

CIGARETTE SMOKING

ACCORDING TO THE U.S. Public Health Service, nicotine addiction is the "most widespread example of drug dependence in our country."

Smoking is the single most preventable cause of premature death and disability in the United States. Every year, 350,000 Americans die prematurely from diseases caused by cigarette smoking such as lung cancer, emphysema, and coronary heart disease. Smoking is also a major risk factor for peripheral vascular disease, which is a narrowing of the blood vessels that carry blood to the arms and legs. If a blood clot blocks an already narrowed artery, an arm or leg could be damaged or lost.

Smoking has also had severe consequences on the nation's economy. Estimated annual healthcare costs for smoking related illness total is at a staggering $76 billion. Workplace smoking related illness in the country accounts for approximately 62% of the total annual healthcare costs with $47 billion.

Many people smoke for years and are not aware of the extent of the damage brought on by their habit. We have serviced clients with calculated smoking histories up to 50,000 total packs. Recent studies show that at 500 total packs a smoker could suffer enough back pain to warrant a consultation. Moreover, studies are starting to define the amount of exposure to cigarette smoke that would cause coronary artery disease, aneurysms, stroke, and cancer.

Associated Unhealthy Lifestyle: Smokers tend to be less active and less fit with decreased lung capacity. Smoker's cough might lead to increased spinal pressure which would exacerbate nerve roots that are already within a tight canal.

Inactivity, itself, is associated with increased rates of back pain.

Packs/ Day	Days/ Year	Years	Pack Years	Total Packs	Risk as defined in the Scientific Literature
1	365	1 year	1	365	Heart attack 500 Packs for significant spine pain
1	365	5 years	5	1,825	Stroke
2	365	5 years	10	3,650	Men over 45 years – bronchogenic carcinoma >60 years old, spiral CT – rule out lung cancer
1	365	10 years	10	3,650	
2	365	10 years	20	7,300	Rheumatoid arthritis
1	365	20 years	20	7,300	
2	365	20 years	40	14,600	Emphysema Pulmonary fibrosis, Follicular lymphoma
1	365	60 years	60	21,900	Rectal and colon cancer

LACK OF BLOOD SUPPLY THEORY

The disc space has a very limited blood supply under normal circumstances. Smoking constricts the artery and cuts off this area without overlapping blood supply (watershed area). Without proper blood supply it is easier for rips and tears of the disc interspace to occur, known as annular tears, which leads to disc degeneration and pain.

POISON THEORY

Cigarette smoking introduces nicotine into the bloodstream and increases the carbon dioxide (CO_2) content of your blood. Both nicotine and CO_2 poison the discs. Since the discs of the spine have less metabolic activity and potential, it makes it easier for an annular tear to occur.

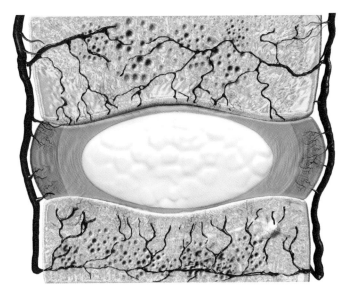

Normal disc with arteries fully open. Even in this optimal condition there is tenuous blood supply of the disc space.

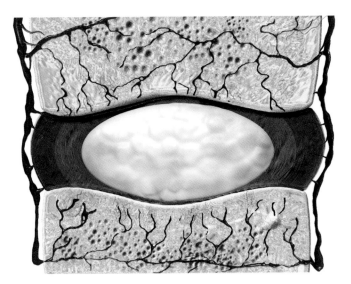

With smoking spinal arteries constrict sending blood to the brain. The normal tenuous blood supply of the disc space is diminished. The disc becomes metabolically poisoned.

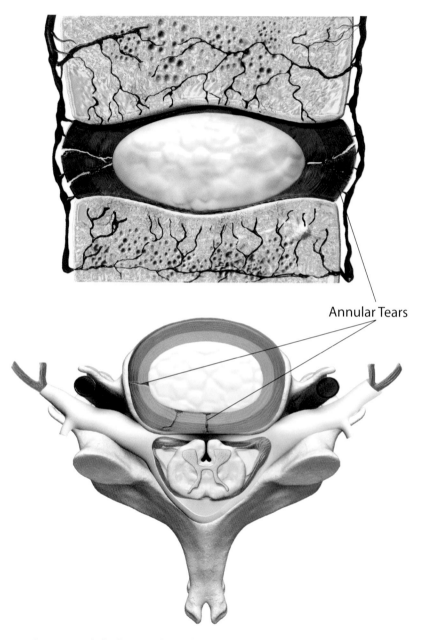

Annular Tears

With time and further smoking the discs crack and rip (**annular tears**), beginning the pathway to disc degeneration and destruction.

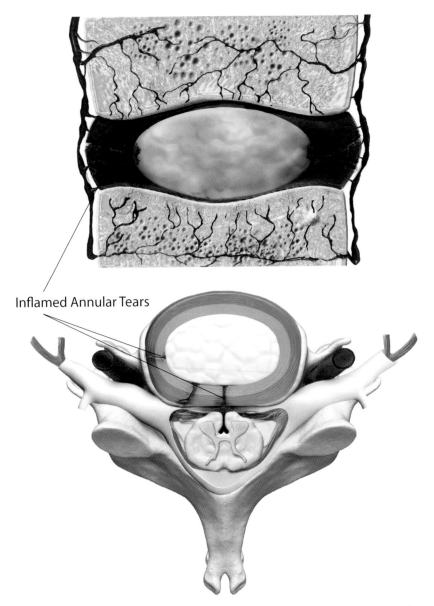

Inflamed Annular Tears

With time and further smoking the discs crack and rip (**annular tears**), beginning the pathway to disc degeneration and destruction, which worsens with the addition of inflammation. Inflammation is a biological response to harmful stimuli. This a process where the body tries to remove and repair the harmful stimulus. Unfortunately, inflammation may lead to further breakdown.

ALCOHOL

SOME STUDIES SUGGEST that moderate alcohol consumption of one drink per day for women and up to two drinks per day for men has been associated with health benefits, such as long-term cognitive protection and reducing the risk of developing heart disease. Other reports do not support these claims and even light to moderate alcohol intake might not benefit everyone. In some cases, the safest choice is to avoid alcohol entirely; the possible benefits do not outweigh the risks of damaging the heart as well as other internal organs.

As a physician, I am careful to make any recommendations, especially those concerning alcohol. Alcohol should only be considered for people as an additional modality for the well-proven, cardiovascular risk-reducing alternatives such as a low-fat diet and exercise. The World Health Organization reports that the harmful use of alcohol results in 2.5 million deaths each year, of which 320,000 are young people between the ages of 15 and 29.

Although red wine is rich in polyphenols (antioxidants that prevent or neutralize the damaging effects of free radicals on healthy cells), which has been shown to have cardio-protective and anti-carcinogenic qualities, many other beverage and food items are as well. Grape juice, green tea, white tea, black tea, coffee, olive oil, and chocolate are all rich in polyphenols, but they also have the benefit of being alcohol-free.

The GDP of the world in 2010 was $62 trillion. The European Union accounted for $16 trillion and the U.S. $14 trillion. The economic burden to the world for alcohol abuse ranged from $2 trillion to $3 trillion.

HISTORY

A comprehensive history of alcohol consumption is taken, including a tally over a specified amount of years. For example, this individual has had 4 ounces of red wine every day for 20 years, totaling 29,220 ounces and approximately 584,000 calories ingested. It is estimated that 3,500 calories will equal 1 pound of weight gained. Over a 20 year span, this individual gained 166 lbs., or about 8 pounds a year.

An increase to 12 ounces of alcohol per day could lead to a lifetime tally of 88,000 ounces consumed and a weight gain of 500 pounds by alcohol alone. Consuming this much alcohol is associated with lack of exercise, and poor nutrition. This could also be associated with significant medical, lifestyle, and emotional problems.

How much alcohol are you consuming? What are the implications for your health? What do you sacrifice in your emotional and personal life, and your well-being?

Alcohol Use	Ounces/ Day	Calories/ Ounce	Years	Total Ounces	Total Calories	Weight Gained in Pounds
Wine	4	20	20	29,120	582,400	166
Wine	12	20	20	87,600	1,752,000	500

	Calories per Ounce
Beer – Regular	10
Gin/Rum/Vodka/Whisky/Tequila/ Brandy/Cognac	65
Liquors	120
Red and White Wine	20
Sweet Wine	25
Cocktails – Martini/Manhattan/ Daiquiri/ Whiskey Sour/Margarita	30 – 40

PRESCRIBED DRUG USE

NARCOTICS ARE WIDELY PRESCRIBED in the U.S. It is considered abuse when narcotics are used to seek feelings of well-being apart from their pain-relief applications. Constituting only 4.6% of the world's population, Americans are responsible for consuming 80% of the global opioid supply, 99% of the global hydrocodone supply, as well as two-thirds of the world's illegal drugs. There are multiple adverse consequences to narcotic use including, but not limited to, hormonal and immune system effects, abuse and addiction, tolerance, and hyperalgesia. Reports have shown that long-term opioid users have increased the overall cost of healthcare, disability, rates of surgery, and late opioid use.

In my opinion, with time and study we could find actual structural neuroplastic changes of the brain with long-term use of narcotics. This engrained degenerative neuroplasticity could, therefore, call for new strategies to help people change their habits. Sadly, in a few cases, early deaths have been observed by friends, family and loved ones of those that persisted with high-level narcotics.

Now, stop and think. How long and how much pain medication have I consumed? What are the long-term manifestations of this intervention?

	Mgs. Used per Day	Days per Year	Years	Total
Hydrocodone		365		
Oxycodone		365		
Oxycontin		365		
Morphine		365		

ILLICIT DRUG USE

A UNITED NATIONS report issued in Stockholm stated that the illegal global drug trade generated an estimated $321.6 billion in 2003, the most recent year for which figures were available. Of that amount, $214 billion, or 67%, of the money was made at the retail level in the streets and back alleys. Of the $214 billion, North America was responsible for 44% of all estimated illicit drug sales and Europe followed with 33%. Africa's illicit drug sales were the lowest at 4%.

Illegal drugs are associated with distinct brain changes seen on MRIs, significant mental sufferings, loss of immunity, prevalence of infections, heart and lung problems, and early death. This lifestyle is not constructive for a fit spinal result. Stated otherwise, long-term use of illicit drugs may predict a lifestyle of pain.

Drugs	Use per Day	Days per Year	Years	Total
Marijuana		365		
Cocaine		365		
Metamphetamine		365		

BIBLIOGRAPHY

SMOKING

Castelli WP. *Diet, smoking, and alcohol: influence on coronary heart disease risk.* Am J Kidney Dis. 1990 Oct;16(4 Suppl 1):41-6.

Cottin V, Brillet PY, Nunes H, Cordier JF; Groupe d'étude et de recherche sur les maladies "orphelines" pulmonaires (GERM"O"P). *[Combined pulmonary fibrosis and emphysema].* Presse Med. 2007 Jun;36(6 Pt 2):936-44. Epub 2007 Apr 18.

Henschke CI, McCauley DI, Yankelevitz DF, Naidich DP, McGuinness G, Miettinen OS, Libby D, Pasmantier M, Koizumi J, Altorki N, Smith JP. *Early lung cancer action project: a summary of the findings on baseline screening.* Oncologist. 2001;6(2):147-52.

Infante M, Lutman FR, Cavuto S, Brambilla G, Chiesa G, Passera E, Angeli E, Chiarenza M, Aranzulla G, Cariboni U, Alloisio M, Incarbone M, Testori A, Destro A, Cappuzzo F, Roncalli M, Santoro A, Ravasi G; DANTE Study Group. *Lung cancer screening with spiral CT: baseline results of the randomized DANTE trial.* Lung Cancer. 2008 Mar;59(3):355-63. Epub 2007 Oct 23.

Kannel WB, Higgins M. *Smoking and hypertension as predictors of cardiovascular risk in population studies.* J Hypertens Suppl. 1990 Sep;8(5):S3-8.

Liang PS, Chen TY, Giovannucci E. *Cigarette smoking and colorectal cancer incidence and mortality: systematic review and meta-analysis.* Int J Cancer. 2009 May 15;124(10):2406-15.

Love BB, Biller J, Jones MP, Adams HP Jr, Bruno A. *Cigarette smoking. A risk factor for cerebral infarction in young adults.* Arch Neurol. 1990 Jun;47(6):693-8.

Mokdad A. H.; Marks, JS; Stroup, DF; Gerberding, JL. *"Actual Causes of Death in the United States, 2000".* JAMA 291 (10): 1238–45, (2004).

Morton LM, Hartge P, Holford TR, Holly EA, Chiu BC, Vineis P, Stagnaro E, Willett EV, Franceschi S, La Vecchia C, Hughes AM, Cozen W, Davis S, Severson RK, Bernstein L, Mayne ST, Dee FR, Cerhan JR, Zheng T. *Cigarette smoking and risk of non-Hodgkin lymphoma: a pooled analysis from the International Lymphoma Epidemiology Consortium (interlymph).* Cancer Epidemiol Biomarkers Prev. 2005 Apr;14(4):925-33.

Mühlhauser I. *Cigarette smoking and diabetes: an update.* Diabet Med. 1994 May;11(4):336-43.

Sugiyama D, Nishimura K, Tamaki K, Tsuji G, Nakazawa T, Morinobu A, Kumagai S. *Impact of smoking as a risk factor for developing rheumatoid arthritis: a meta-analysis of observational studies.* Ann Rheum Dis. 2010 Jan;69(1):70-81.

WHO Report on the Global Tobacco Epidemic, 2010. Geneva: World Health Organization. 2010.

Wisnivesky JP, Szwarcberg JB, McGinn TG. *Lung cancer. Screening, counseling, and treating long-term smokers.* Geriatrics. 2002 Nov;57(11):28-32.

ALCOHOL

Beulens JW, Rimm EB, Ascherio A, Spiegelman D, Hendriks HF, Mukamal KJ. *Alcohol consumption and risk for coronary heart disease among men with hypertension.* Ann Intern Med. 2007 Jan 2;146(1):10-9.

Mukamal KJ, Chiuve SE, Rimm EB. *Alcohol consumption and risk for coronary heart disease in men with healthy lifestyles.* Arch Intern Med. 2006 Oct 23;166(19):2145-50.

Sinkiewicz W, Weglarz M. *Alcohol and wine and cardiovascular diseases in epidemiologic studies.* Przegl Lek. 2009;66(5):233-8.

DRUG USE

Geibprasert S, Gallucci M, Krings T. *Addictive illegal drugs: structural neuroimaging.* AJNR Am J Neuroradiol. 2010 May;31(5):803-8. Epub 2009 Oct 29.

Hoshi R, Mullins K, Boundy C, Brignell C, Piccini P, Curran HV. *Neurocognitive function in current and ex-users of ecstasy in comparison to both matched polydrug-using controls and drug-naïve controls.* Psychopharmacology (Berl). 2007 Oct;194(3):371-9. Epub 2007 Jul 1.

Iyalomhe GB. *Cannabis abuse and addiction: a contemporary literature review.* Niger J Med. 2009 Apr-Jun;18(2):128-33.

Khalsa JH, Treisman G, McCance-Katz E, Tedaldi E. *Medical consequences of drug abuse and co-occurring infections: research at the National Institute on Drug Abuse.* Subst Abus. 2008;29(3):5-16.

Rogers G, Elston J, Garside R, Roome C, Taylor R, Younger P, Zawada A, Somerville M. *The harmful health effects of recreational ecstasy: a systematic review of observational evidence.* Health Technol Assess. 2009 Jan;13(6):iii-iv, ix-xii, 1-315.

Vroegop MP, Franssen EJ, van der Voort PH, van den Berg TN, Langeweg RJ, Kramers C. *The emergency care of cocaine intoxications.* Neth J Med. 2009 Apr;67(4):122-6.

CHAPTER 8

Wholesome Options

FOOD CONSIDERATIONS

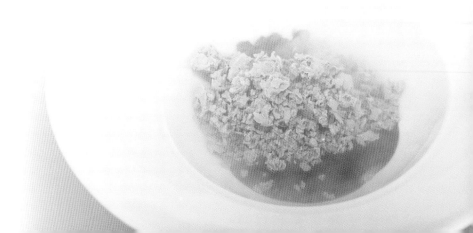

Every morsel of food consumed should do the body good...

HIGH OCTANE
VS. LOW OCTANE FUEL

STARTING YOUR DAY with a cup of coffee and a pastry is similar to filling a Ferrari with low-octane fuel.

Be especially thoughtful with your first meal. Start your day with a high-protein, low-glycemic breakfast or shake.

High-protein meals, at any point in the day, will provide long-term energy and help prevent cravings and energy crashes. Simple-carbohydrate meals, on the other hand, briefly fill and satisfy you and enhances your cravings to eat, and eat, and eat. (*Special thanks to Ahmed Al-Khawanky for modeling this scenario.*)

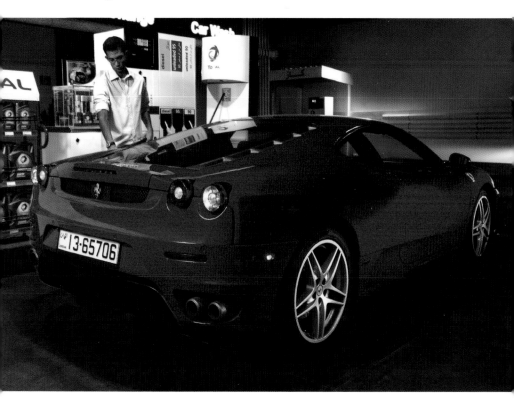

THE MEANING OF FOOD

The primary role of food is fuel for the body. However, food can carry different meanings to different people.

When I was a young boy, my mother would return from the grocery store with a Cadbury milk chocolate bar just for me. Till this day, I associate a Cadbury bar with the love of mom. What are the emotional connections to the foods you eat?

THE EMOTIONAL COMPONENT

In many modern societies it is easy to overeat. All kinds of foods are, readily, within our reach in the form of fast food establishments, packaged snacks, and candies and cakes, etc.

Many people go through each week planning their work schedule or weekend recreation but fail to take the time to schedule nutritious, portioned meals. Most people would rather routinely service and take care of their cars than their own bodies.

Being unplanned with nutrition and feeling sad or depressed could be a destructive combination. Add the probability of poor sleep and it is at these times that people make poor choices and reach for comfort foods, which could lead to weight gain.

Many people grab food habitually and are completely unaware of the addiction that has developed. The body will go through withdrawals from sugar much in the same way it goes through withdrawals from nicotine or caffeine. Someone withdrawing from sugar will most likely experience nausea and irritability.

THE INSULIN COMPONENT

Carbohydrates are listed as simple or complex. Classification of a food depends on its chemical structure and how rapidly the sugar is digested and absorbed.

Elevated sugar levels in the blood is a sign the body has more than it needs. The body is not burning the sugar so it accumulates. Insulin is released to take that sugar and store it as glycogen, but the body stores very little glycogen at one time. Once filled, additional sugar in the blood spikes insulin levels and the sugar is stored as saturated fat. The rapid breakdown of simple, and even complex, carbohydrates leads to hunger, which usually leads to more carbohydrate consumption, which creates a damaging cycle that increases the risk of obesity.

Thirty to forty-five minutes before medium to high-carbohydrate meals, have a low fat, low carbohydrate protein shake. Protein slows the breakdown of carbohydrates, which prevents spikes of insulin.

Simple carbohydrates have single (monosaccharide) or double (disaccharide) sugars, while complex carbohydrates contain three or more sugars.

Complex carbohydrates, often referred to as "starchy" carbs, include foods such as legumes, whole grain breads, and most vegetables.

Simple carbohydrates that contain naturally occurring vitamins and minerals include fruits and fruit juices, milk and milk products, honey, and certain vegetables.

WORLD CLASS SCHEDULING

I recommend planning daily foods and scheduling them as though planning for a world-class athlete. This would include eating 6 small, healthful meals to keep blood sugar levels in normal range and to keep the metabolism burning efficiently.

Begin the day with 8–16 ounces of water and schedule a total of at least 64 ounces of fluid per day (most of which should be water), and up to 128 ounces if athletic or a physical laborer in hot climates.

Skim milk is a great source of Vitamin D.

A multiple vitamin and mineral supplement should be considered to cover the body's requirements (not FDA minimum standards) for optimal health and prevent deficiencies.

LAYERING

LAYERING A CUP OF COFFEE demonstrates the importance of keeping an eye on the finishing. A cup of black coffee has 2 calories; with sugar, 12 calories; with sugar and milk, 30 calories; with sugar and half and half, 60 calories; and with sugar, half and half, and whipped cream, at least 160 calories.

	Amount	Calories
Whip cream	1 oz.	100
1 Half and Half Cream	2 containers = 1 oz.	40
Whole Milk	1 oz.	17
2% Milk	1 oz.	14
White Sugar	1 tsp.	10
Brown Sugar	1tsp.	11
Coffee	6ozs.	2

10 Great Food Options	10 Poor Choices
Water	Soda
Vegetables	Processed food
Fruits	Candy, Confection
Nuts	Pastry
Eggs	Processed meats
Lean Meats and Fish	Dark meat
Dairy: Low-fat cheese and milk, yogurt	High calorie mixed drinks and coffees
Whole grain pasta	White pasta
Whole grain bread	White bread
Brown rice	White rice
Sugar options: Agave, Honey	White sugar

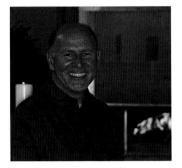

C ARLO CITERA, restauranteur of the Cosimo's restaurant group in Poughkeepsie, New York, is a great proponent of serving colorful, bountiful fresh vegetables. Roasted vegetables are a delicious, healthy option any time of the day. Roasted vegetables may be served with a balsamic vinaigrette dressing. Organic vegetables provide vitamins, minerals and fibers. My favorite dish is a roasted vegetable wrap with jalapeno peppers.

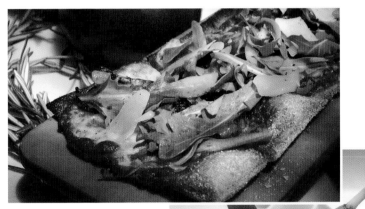

Carlo's group makes an exceptional gluten-free flat crusted pizza with minimal cheese and generous servings of fresh vegetables.

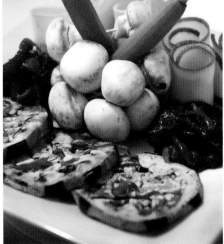

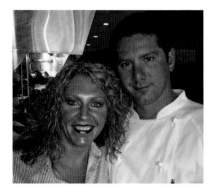

T HOMAS AND BECKY Kacherski are proprietors of Crew Restaurant of Poughkeepsie, New York. Crew offers a pan roasted organic chicken breast with truffled potato croquettes, seasonal vegetables and a mushroom Marsala sauce, which is simply exquisite.

Organic foods are foods that are certified by the Organic Foods Production Act of 1990 to respond to site-specific conditions by integrating cultural, biological, and mechanical practices that foster cycling of resources, promote ecological balance, and conserve biodiversity. These foods are produced using methods that do not include pesticides, chemical fertilizers, genetically modified organisms, and are not processed with irradiation, industrial solvents, or chemical food additives.

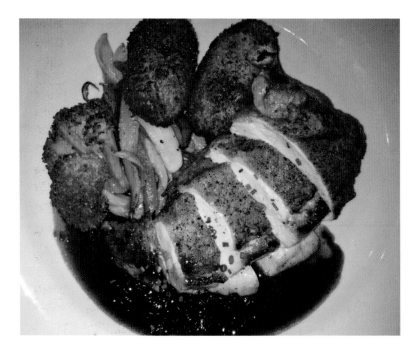

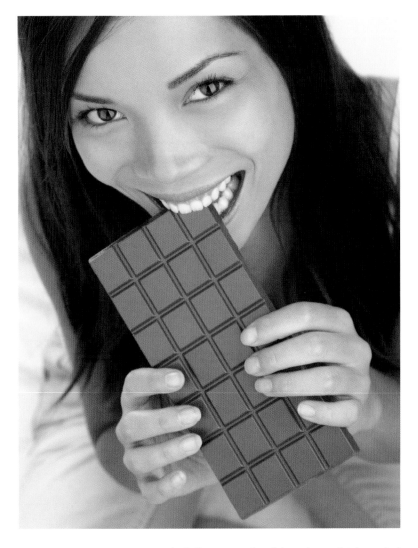

In 2001 Americans consumed 3 billion pounds of chocolate, which totaled $14 billion in sales. This averaged to 12 lbs./year per person, consisting of: 27000 calories, 1530 g fat, 1130 mg cholesterol, 4400 mg sodium, 3150 g carbs, 350 g protein. The average Swiss national consumed 22 lbs. of chocolate; Austrian, 20; Irish, 20; German, 18; and Norwegian, 20. Twenty-two percent of chocolate consumption occurs between 8pm and mid-night. Consumption is highest during the winter months.

SAVORING

CHEF ANTHONY GONCALVES of 42 The Restaurant in White Plains, New York, states, "The Black Forest dessert is a way for me to bring part of the creative processes behind my menu right into the dining room. I add liquid nitrogen to a chocolate cream to make "pebbles" of ice cream on the spot. I've decided to serve this

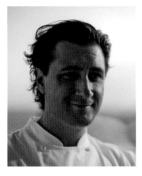

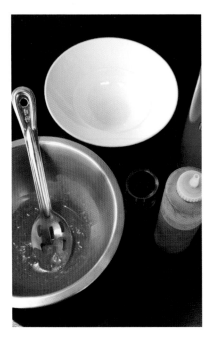

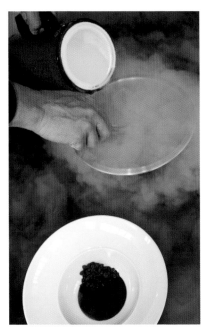

over the cherry "brook" to touch on the sweet tooth of chocolate and fruit lovers alike. What I love about this dessert is that the unique temperature and texture allows my guests to enjoy a smaller portion and less sugar. The flavors and presentation make for a memorable finale to the meal."

CHERRY BROOK	CHOCOLATE CREAM
Fresh cherry purée	Milk
Simple almond extract	Cream
	Bittersweet chocolate

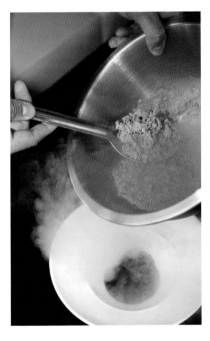
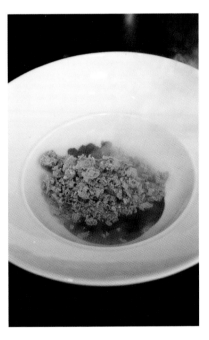

VITAMINS AND SUPPLEMENTS

I RECOMMEND a multivitamin a day for my patients. A vitamin B complex per day might help reduce or eliminate neuropathic or nerve pain. There is some evidence that Omega-3 could play a stabilizing role on nerves. Glucosamine and chondroitin sulfate have been shown to play a role in the metabolism of hip, knee and facet joints.

Risk of breast cancer, colon cancer, pancreatic cancer, and ovarian cancer have all been significantly reduced by 1000 international units or 25 micrograms of vitamin D. The National Health and Nutrition Examination Survey concluded that low levels of vitamin D (<17.8 ng/ml) was independently associated with an increase of all cause mortality in the general population. However, increased mortality was also found in those with higher concentrations of vitamin D (>50 ng/ml). Excess or deficiency in the Vitamin D system appear to cause abnormal functioning and premature aging. How much vitamin D is enough? The American Academy of Orthopedic Surgeons and recent research support that the body needs at least 1000 international units per day for good health – depending on age, weight and growth. In general, babies (especially mothers who are breastfeeding) and small children should intake at least 400 IU of Vitamin D daily. Children over age 5, adolescents, and adults should get a minimum of 1000 IU of Vitamin D each day. Check with your medical doctor to assess your levels by blood test.

Since they dissolve in fat, vitamins A, D, E, and K are known as fat-soluble vitamins. These fat-soluble vitamins are absorbed from the small intestine along with dietary fat. Fat malabsorption resulting from various diseases such as cystic fibrosis, Crohn's disease, and ulcerative colitis is associated with poor absorption of these vitamins. Primarily stored in the liver and adipose (fatty) tissue, fat-soluble vitamins are generally excreted more slowly than their water-soluble counterparts, vitamins B and C.

Vitamin A and D can accumulate in the body and have toxic

effects when taken in very high doses for prolonged periods of time. For example, The Nurses Health Study looked at 72,337 postmenopausal women over an 18 year period and found that women whose daily intake was 10,000 international units (IU), or 3,000 micrograms (mcg), per day as retinol equivalents were 48% more likely to have a hip fracture.

High doses of retinol, one of the animal forms of vitamin A, might interfere with the activity of vitamin D, a vitamin that facilitates the absorption of calcium.

Worldwide, more than 50% of the population is vitamin D deficient. If you shun the sun, have milk allergies, or follow a strict vegetarian or vegan diet, you might be at risk for vitamin D deficiency.

Low blood levels of vitamin D have been associated with increased risk of death from cardiovascular disease, severe asthma in children, cognitive impairment, and cancer.

Research suggests that vitamin D could play a role in the prevention and treatment of type1(juvenile) and type2 (adult onset) diabetes, hypertension, glucose intolerance and multiple sclerosis.

The conclusion that vitamin D has the potential to prevent cancer lies in its role in a wide range of cellular mechanisms that are central to the development of cancer. These effects can be mediated through vitamin D receptors that are expressed in cancer cells. The risk of breast cancer, colon cancer, pancreatic cancer, and ovarian cancer have been significantly reduced by ingesting 1000 IU, or 25 mcg, of vitamin D per day.

Calcium	Recommended
Males and females 9 to 18 years	1,300 mg per day
Women and men 19 to 50 years	1,000 mg per day
Pregnant or nursing women up to age 18	1,300 mg per day
Pregnant or nursing women 19 to 50 years	1,000 mg per day
Women and men over 50	1,200 mg per day

Food	Amount	Calcium (in mg)
Yogurt, plain, low fat	8 oz	415
Skim milk	1 cup	306
Spinach, frozen, boiled	1 cup	291
Yogurt, plain, whole milk	8 oz	275
Cheese food, pasteurized American	1 oz	162
Cottage cheese, 1% milk fat	1 cup	138
Baked beans, canned	1 cup	154

In the 2008 Selenium and Vitamin E Cancer Prevention Trial (SELECT), the study concluded that, whether taken alone or together, Vitamin E and Selenium (a trace mineral) were not effective in the prevention of prostate cancer. The data also suggested that the vitamin/trace mineral combination wouldn't produce a 25% reduction in prostate cancer.

Between the four groups involved in the SELECT study, there were no significant differences, statistically, in the rates of prostate cancer. There was a higher instance of prostate cancer in the group of men that supplemented with only vitamin E. This does not in itself suggest that vitamin E is a cause of prostate cancer and these differences could have occurred solely by chance.

Sometimes supplementation can lead to adverse outcomes. In the Selenium and Vitamin E Cancer Prevention Trial (SELECT) statistically non-significant increased risks of prostate cancer with vitamin E alone [relative risk (RR) = 1.13, P = 0.06) and newly diagnosed Type 2 diabetes mellitus with selenium alone (RR = 1.07, P = 0.16) were observed.

SUGAR

SIMPLE CARBOHYDRATES are found in processed and refined sugar products like candy; non-diet carbonated beverages such as soda; syrups and, of course, table sugar. White rice, flour, and potatoes are other common examples.

Simple sugars that are stripped of their naturally occurring nutrients such as vitamins, minerals, and fiber are often referred to as "empty calories." These refined sugars provide only calories and can lead to weight gain.

Four classes of simple sugars; sucrose, fructose, honey, and malts are deemed by most health professionals and nutritionists as "harmful" to optimal health when consumption is prolonged in amounts above 15% of the total calories derived from carbohydrates.

Some might be surprised to find honey on the above list. Although honey is a natural sweetener, it has 65 calories per tablespoon compared to the 48 calories per tablespoon in table sugar. Honey also causes greater incidents of tooth decay than table sugar.

The best option is to limit or remove sweeteners such as table sugar and honey.

GLYCEMIC INDEX

The glycemic index is a ranking system for carbohydrates according to their effect on our blood glucose levels. Low glycemic index carbs produce only small fluctuations in our blood glucose and insulin levels. This is the secret to diminishing risks for heart disease, diabetes and is a key driver for weight loss.

Low glycemic index options include breakfast cereals based on oats; steel cut oats; barley and bran; fruits and vegetables; salad, especially with vinaigrette dressing and nuts; and fructose sugar.

Medium glycemic index options include breads with true wholegrains, or stone-ground brown flour, brown rice, basmati rice, whole wheat pasta, noodles, and quinoa.

High glycemic index options include baked potatoes, watermelon, white bread, white pasta, most white rice, most breakfast cereals, white sugar, glucose and maltose sugars.

Sugar	Ounces/Day	Years	Total
Consumed	4	1	1,460 ounces 91 pounds
Consumed	4	20	29,200 ounces 1,825 pounds

BOWEL MOTILITY

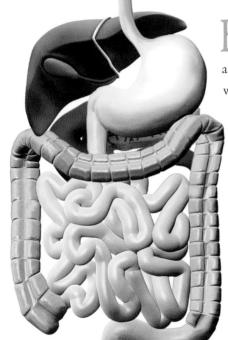

BOWEL MOTILITY and movements are critical in all aspects of life and are key to spinal well-being. The body is wired to have a bowel movement in the morning, although it is capable of having them at any time during the day.

Gastrointestinal symptoms such as diarrhea or constipation are prevalent among shift workers and flight travelers that change time zones. Both are examples of disruptions in biological rhythms. Narcotics will delay and inhibit bowel movements, while a diet high in fiber will improve movements. Caffeine is a mild diuretic and excessive intake draws fluid away from the stool, making them difficult to pass. However, 1-2 cups of coffee in the morning has been shown to increase the chance of a successful bowel movement.

As a spine specialist, I have helped many patients by suggesting they be conscious of their bowel movements. I believe that decreasing the intra-abdominal load mechanically leads to decreased pressure on the nerves. The body and the spine, in particular, might be helped chemically by diminishing this load. Fruits, vegetables and fibers improve bowel motility.

BIBLIOGRAPHY

VITAMINS AND SUPPLEMENTS

Cabanillas F. *Vitamin C and cancer: what can we conclude--1,609 patients and 33 years later?* P R Health Sci J. 2010 Sep;29(3):215-7. University of Puerto Rico School of Medicine, San Juan, Puerto Rico. fcabanil@mdanderson.org.

Chung M, Balk EM, Brendel M, Ip S, Lau J, Lee J, Lichtenstein A, Patel K, Raman G, Tatsioni A, Terasawa T, Trikalinos TA. *Vitamin D and calcium: a systematic review of health outcomes.* Evid Rep Technol Assess (Full Rep). 2009 Aug;(183):1-420.

Clarke R, Halsey J, Lewington S, Lonn E, Armitage J, Manson JE, Bønaa KH, Spence JD, Nygård O, Jamison R, Gaziano JM, Guarino P, Bennett D, Mir F, Peto R, Collins R; B-Vitamin Treatment Trialists' Collaboration. *Effects of lowering homocysteine levels with B vitamins on cardiovascular disease, cancer, and cause-specific mortality: Meta-analysis of 8 randomized trials involving 37 485 individuals.* Arch Intern Med. 2010 Oct 11;170(18):1622-31.

Dunn BK, Richmond ES, Minasian LM, Ryan AM, Ford LG. *A nutrient approach to prostate cancer prevention: The Selenium and Vitamin E Cancer Prevention Trial (SELECT).* Nutr Cancer. 2010 Oct;62(7):896-918.

Gennari C. *Calcium and vitamin D nutrition and bone disease of the elderly.* Public Health Nutr. 2001 Apr;4(2B):547-59.

Gröber U. *[Vitamin D – an old vitamin in a new perspective].* Med Monatsschr Pharm. 2010 Oct;33(10):376-83.

Ingraham, BA; Bragdon, B; Nohe, A (January 2008). *Molecular basis of the potential of vitamin D to prevent cancer.* Current Medical Research and Opinion 24 (1): 139–49.

Karakuła H, Opolska A, Kowal A, Domański M, Płotka A, Perzyński J. *[Does diet affect our mood? The significance of folic acid and homocysteine].* Pol Merkur Lekarski. 2009 Feb;26(152):136-41.

McGregor GP, Biesalski HK. *Rationale and impact of vitamin C in clinical nutrition.* Curr Opin Clin Nutr Metab Care. 2006 Nov;9(6):697-703.

Melamed, M. L.; Michos, E. D.; Post, W.; Astor, B. (2008). *25-Hydroxyvitamin D Levels and the Risk of Mortality in the General Population.* Archives of Internal Medicine 168 (15): 1629–37.

Pierrot-Deseilligny C, Souberbielle JC. *Is hypovitaminosis D one of the environmental risk factors for multiple sclerosis?* Brain. 2010 Jul;133(Pt 7):1869-88.

Selhub J, Troen A, Rosenberg IH. *B vitamins and the aging brain.* Nutr Rev. 2010 Dec;68 Suppl 2:S112-8. doi: 10.1111/j.1753-4887.2010.00346.x.

Sen CK, Khanna S, Rink C, Roy S. *Tocotrienols: the emerging face of natural vitamin E.* Vitam Horm. 2007;76:203-61.

Toner CD, Davis CD, Milner JA. *The vitamin D and cancer conundrum: aiming at a moving target.* J Am Diet Assoc. 2010 Oct;110(10):1492-500.

Zittermann A. *The estimated benefits of vitamin D for Germany.* Mol Nutr Food Res. 2010 Aug;54(8):1164-71.

CHAPTER 9

Aerobic Activities

THE MORE THAT YOU DO,
THE MORE YOU CAN DO.

THE MORE THE FACET JOINTS
AND NERVES START MOVING,
THE BETTER YOU WILL FEEL.

AIR

AEROBIC ACTIVITIES are mission critical to a healthy functional spine. Aerobic activities with its incorporated deep breathing serve to improve the motion of the spinal segments, motion of the spinal cord, motion of the nerve roots, and it increases the cerebrospinal fluid motion and distribution.

Aerobic activities could also decrease the swelling of the deranged joint and possibly the nerve root. This activity will enhance the range of motion of all joints, especially the facet joints. Aerobic activities lead to improved disc hydration and osmotic motion, which brings more oxygen and nutrition to the area and helps healing factors to the disc and joints arrive at the site in higher quantities.

Aerobic activities increase the lymphatic flow, helping aid the inflammatory response. The lymphatic system is a separate system from arteries and veins. It transports immune cells to and from the lymph nodes.

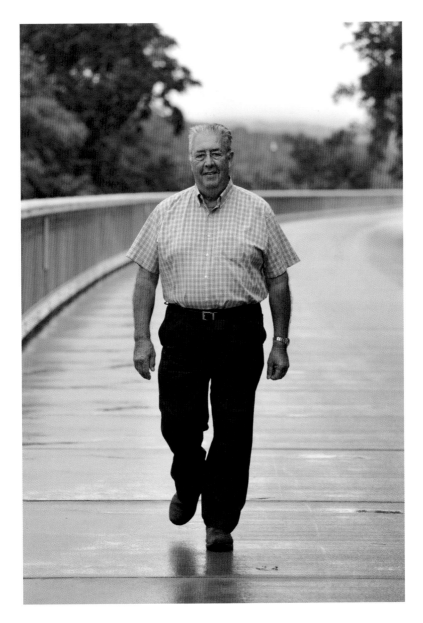

Walking in all forms is beneficial. Walking promotes mental clarity, involves use of the heart and lungs, promotes facet joint mobility and nerve root mobility and function.

Special thanks to Gregory James Chiaramonte, M.D.

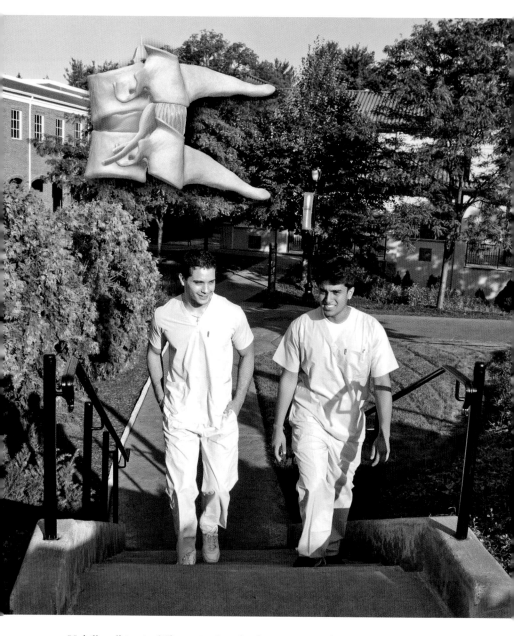

Uphill walking is different in that the facets are in a flexed open position and they might be helpful in conditions where there is nerve root tightness.

Special thanks to Jose Peres and Shawn Jindal

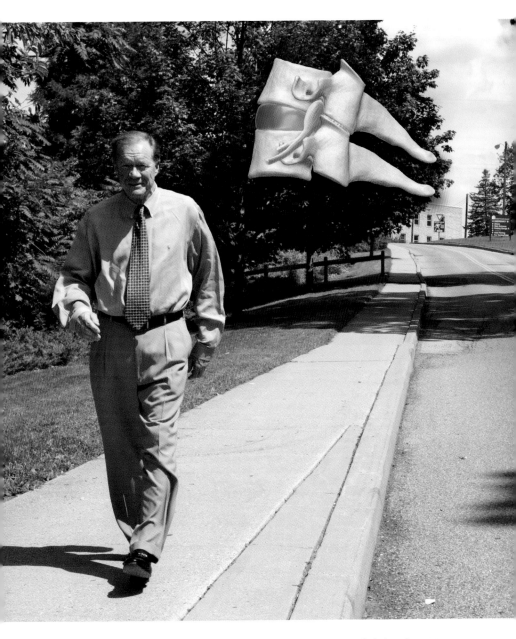

Downhill walking is different in that the facets are in an extended closed position and they could worsen conditions where there is already nerve root tightness.

Special thanks to Robert Savage

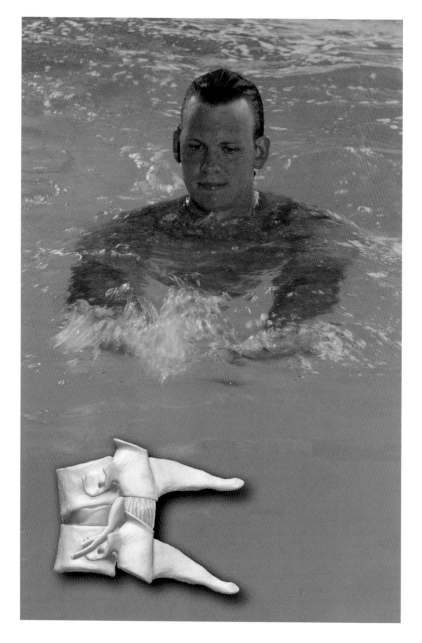

The crawl in swimming is a flexion-based exercise. The facets are in the flexed position with the neuroforamen open, which allows the nerve roots more space. This technique might be helpful in conditions with nerve root tightness.

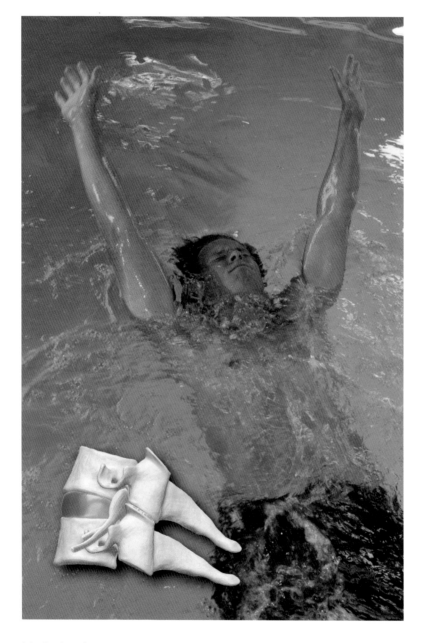

The backstroke in swimming is an extension-based exercise. The facets are in the extended position with the neuroforamen more closed, which gives the nerve roots less space. This technique could exacerbate conditions with nerve root tightness.

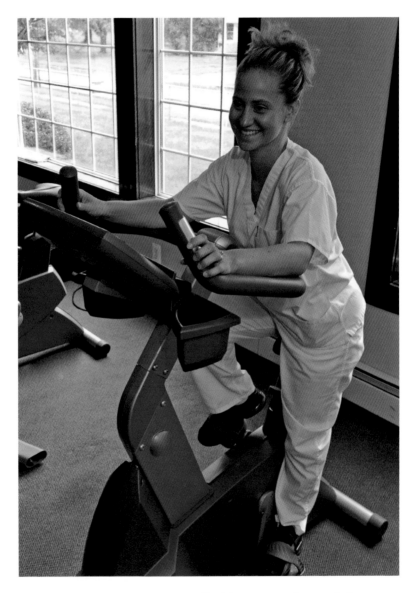

Stationary bike riding is a great way of building your aerobic metabolism.

The height of your seat will determine the posture of your spine. The higher the seat, the more flexion your spine will exhibit. The lower your seat, the more you move into extension of the spine.

Remember to enjoy your ride!

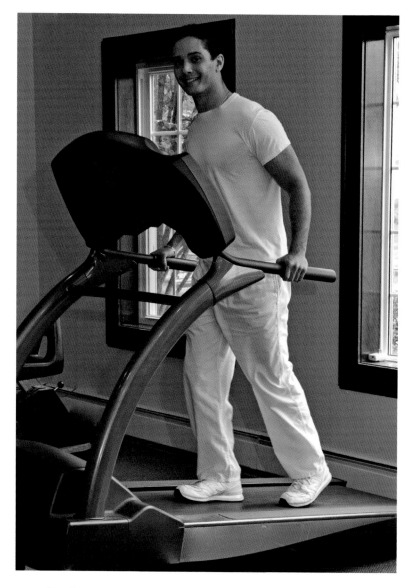

One of my favorite aerobic activities is the rapid incline treadmill. Slowly walking on the edge of a treadmill machine at 45 degrees with your spine straight, for example, will allow you to easily achieve elevated heart rates with minimal motion. This could be an excellent strategy if you are starting to walk through your back or neck pain.

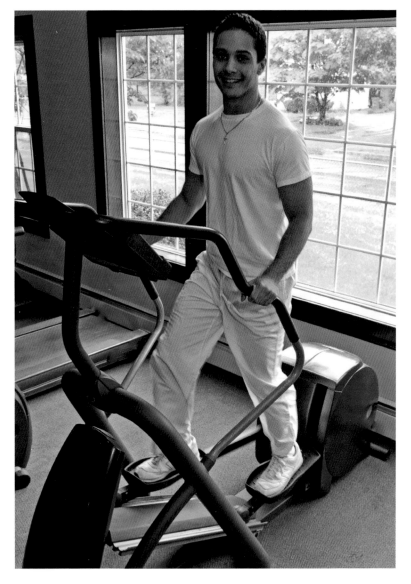

Of aerobic activities, the elliptical cross-trainer offers the least amount of impact to the joints. Keep in mind that there are two true joints called facet joints at every level of the spine. Newer versions of the elliptical cross-trainer simulate running quite well.

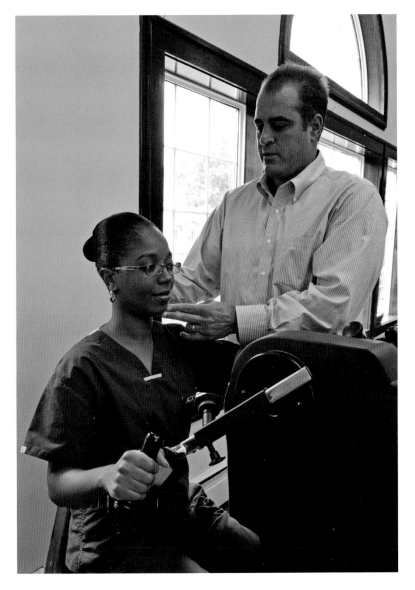

The Upper Body Ergonometer produces variable resistance at fixed speeds. Muscles are loaded to full capability throughout the range of motion.

In rehabiliation of the cervical spine, the physical therapist will work with you to keep proper posture.

Special thanks to Jacqueline Reeder and Christian Campilii, P.T.

CHAPTER 10

Physical Treatments

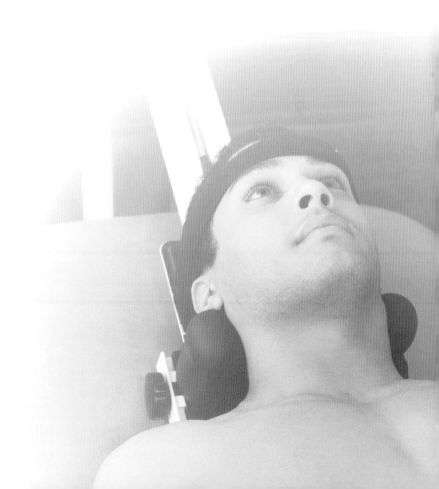

MASSAGES

MASSAGE IS A MANUAL TECHNIQUE of the application of pressure and motion to the soft tissues of the body. Skin, muscles, tendons, and ligaments are improved by encouraging the flow of blood and lymph, which removes tension and restores normal function.

Research sponsored by the National Center for Complementary and Alternative Medicine, a division of the National Institutes of Health, found that a single session of massage caused significant biological changes. Volunteers that received Swedish massage experienced significant decreases in levels of the stress hormone cortisol in blood and saliva, and in arginine vasopressin, a hormone that can lead to increases in cortisol. They also had increases in the number of white blood cells, known as lymphocytes, which are part of the immune system.

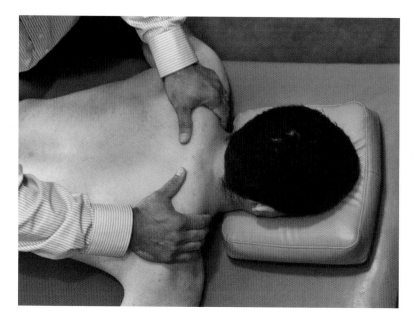

PHYSICAL AGENTS

PHYSICAL AGENTS are techniques and modalities that are employed to physically diminish inflammation and restore function. The advantages of using these modalities include being simple, readily available, and that they are usually medication free. Guidelines must be followed, however, because there may be dangers.

Heat in any fashion might be good for you. While heat and cold are both therapeutic, one has to be careful of use with compromised skin if, for example, there is no feeling. Unfortunately discoloration of skin and burns could, possibly, occur. Please check with your physician or use a licensed physical therapist before employing the agents.

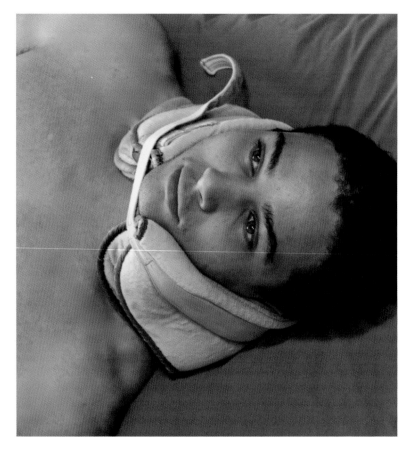

Hot packs are a good way to provide heat that diminishes inflammation and relieves pain. Be careful and use many layers of insulation.

PLEASE DO NOT USE IF YOU HAVE COMPROMISED SKIN INTEGRITY OR SENSATION. This is the most frequent cause of burns in physical therapy.

Total treatment time should be less than 30 minutes. Heat increases blood flow to the local area, bringing nutrients and inflammatory factors. By products and tissue debris are removed.

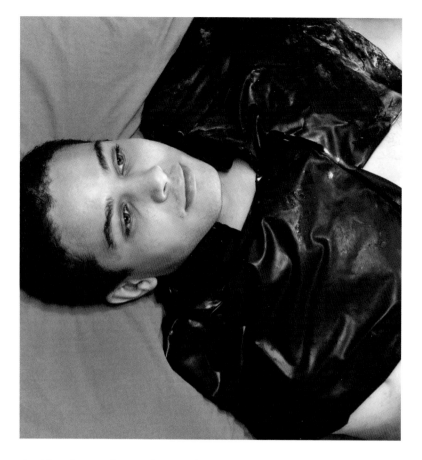

A cold pack is another good way to diminish inflammation and relieve pain.

PLEASE DO NOT USE IF YOU HAVE COMPROMISED SKIN INTEGRITY OR SENSATION.

Total treatment time should be less than 30 minutes. Cold may be applied for relief of pain, and muscle spasm, control of inflammation and swelling. Cold treatments are not recommended with cold intolerance, arterial or sensation impairments.

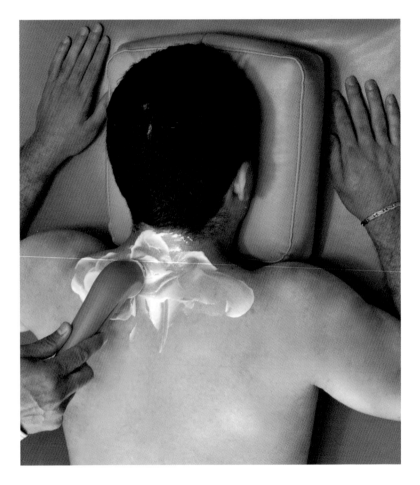

Ultrasound uses acoustic vibrations with frequencies above the audible range. This treatment produces an electrical current with vibration, ultimately producing heat. This treatment should be performed by a licensed therapist only. Ultrasound could utilize steroid cream for diminishing inflammation.

It is *not* recommended near the eyes, brain, reproductive organs, pacemakers, laminectomy sites, malignancy, skeletal immaturity or joint replacements.

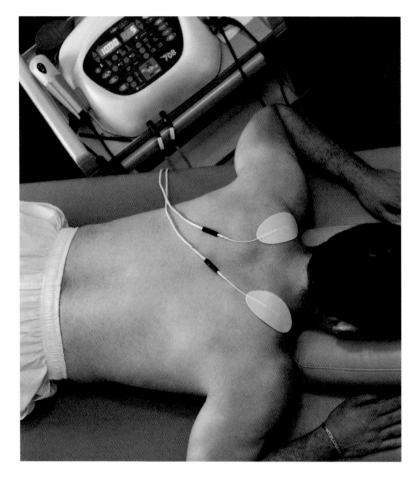

Electrotherapy refers to the therapeutic use of electricity to stimulate nerve or muscle.

Electrotherapy causes muscle group contraction, and increased circulation. Electrotherapy also modifies pain via release of endorphins as well as modifying large A fibers stimulation, diminishing pain.

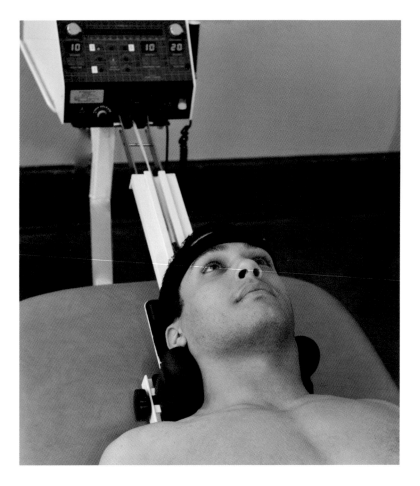

Cervical traction provides a distractive force which serves to provide space in the neuroforamen and compressed nerve roots, especially.

Activities such as walking, standing, and sitting all serve to place a compressive load on the cervical spine. Many patients respond well to cervical traction therapy. Relief of headaches is commonly reported as well.

BIBLIOGRAPHY

MASSAGES

JRapaport MH, Schettler P, Bresee C. *A Preliminary Study of the Effects of a Single Session of Swedish Massage on Hypothalamic-Pituitary-Adrenal and Immune Function in Normal Individuals.* Altern Complement Med. 2010 Sep 1.

CHAPTER 11

Cervical Stabilization

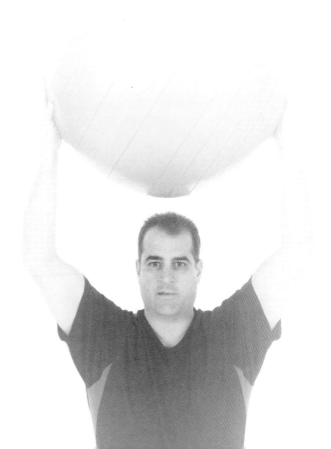

CERVICAL STABILIZATION

CERVICAL STABILIZATION is a process of exercises that focuses on the strengthening of the core muscles of the neck and the proper alignment of the neck. This process serves to rehabilitate and prevent neck injuries

Neutral spine is the proper alignment of the body between postural extremes in its most balanced position. Keep in mind that the spine is not straight. It has curves in the cervical (neck), thoracic (mid-back) and lumbar (lower back) regions. Neutral spine serves to diminish the stress that facet joints, spinal cord, nerve roots, vertebrae and muscles see. It is the most efficient position.

The first layer of exercises uses range of motion of the neck in three planes:

1) Flexion/extension exercises
2) Right and left side rotation
3) Right and left side bending

Patients usually immediately experience an increase in range of motion in this neutral position.

BAD POSTURE

POSTURE describes the attitude or position of the body in space. Understanding posture is critical to the rehabilitation of the cervical spine, and living a pain-free life.

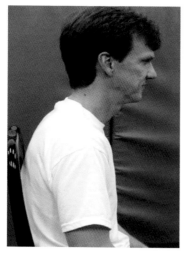

Head Tilted Forward

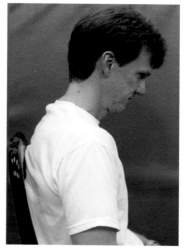

Cervical Kyphosis

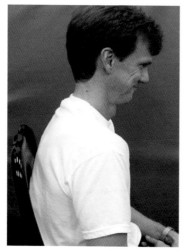

Rounded Shoulder

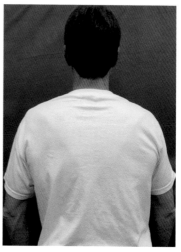

Protracted Scapula

GOOD POSTURE

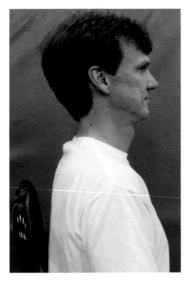

Head Over Shoulder

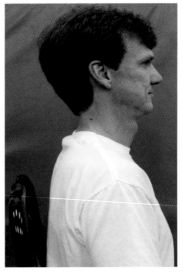

Cervical Lordosis

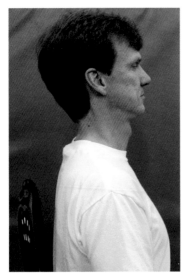

Squared Shoulder

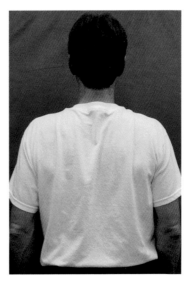

Retracted Scapula

FLEXION/EXTENSION RANGE OF MOTION EXERCISES

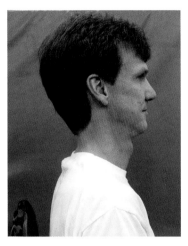

Neutral position is in between
flexion and extension.

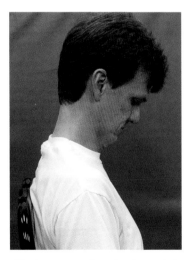

Flexion range of motion is carried
out by bending the neck forward.

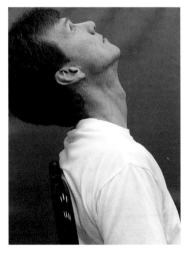

Extension range of motion
is carried out by bending the
neck backward.

SIDE ROTATIONAL RANGE OF MOTION EXERCISES

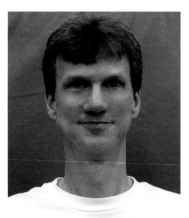

Neutral

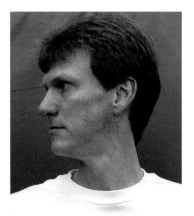

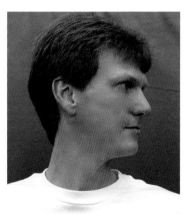

Right rotation range of motion is carried out by rotating the neck towards the right.

Left rotation range of motion is carried out by rotating the neck towards the left.

SIDE BENDING RANGE OF MOTION EXERCISES

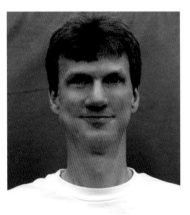

Neutral

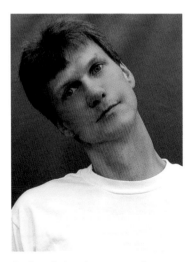

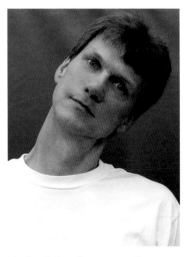

Right side bending range of motion is carried out by bending the neck outwards to the right.

Left side bending range of motion is carried out by bending the neck outwards to the left.

STRENGTHENING

WHEN THE PAIN is better, and range of motion improves, then attention is placed on progressive strengthening:

1	Isometric
2	Gravity Resisted Isometric
3	Pectoralis Muscle Stretching & Strengthening
4	Light Weights
5	Therapeutic Bands

ISOMETRIC STRENGTHENING EXERCISES

FLEXION-BASED isometric exercise is carried out by placing the palm on the front of the head. Resistance is created by pushing the head against the palm of the hand.

◄

Extension-based isometric exercise is carried out by placing the palm on the back of the head. Resistance is created by pushing the head against the palm of the hand. ▼

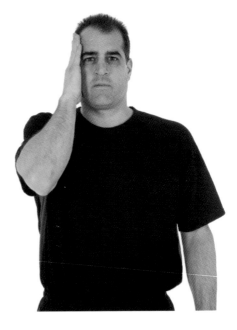

Right side bending-based isometric exercise is carried out by placing the palm on the side of the head. Resistance is created by pushing the head downwards against the palm of the hand.

Left- side bending-based isometric exercise is carried out by placing the palm on the side of the head. Resistance is created by pushing the head downwards against the palm of the hand.

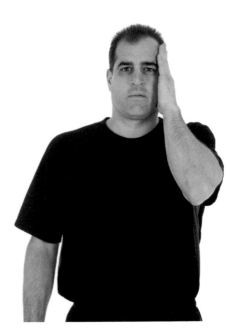

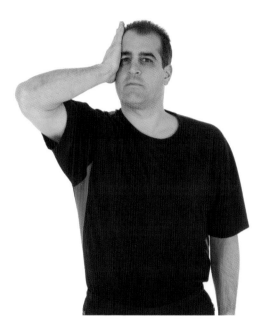

Right side rotation-based isometric exercise is carried out by placing the palm on the side of the head. Resistance is created by rotating the head outwards against the palm of the hand.

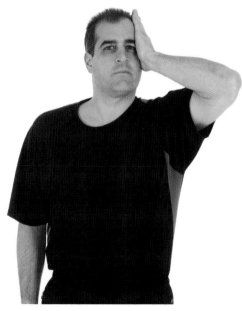

Left side rotation-based isometric exercise is carried out by placing the palm on the side of the head. Resistance is created by rotating the head outwards against the palm of the hand.

GRAVITY RESISTED ISOMETRIC EXERCISES

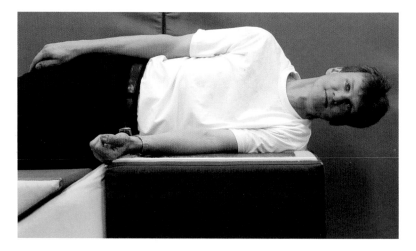

Side bending gravity resisted isometric exercise is carried out by lying on a surface with the neck free.

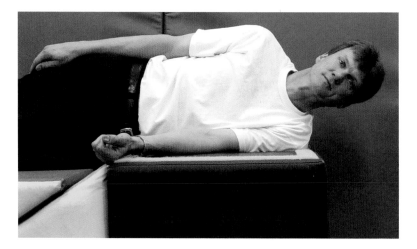

Strengthening in the side bending position is achieved by bending the neck towards the shoulder.

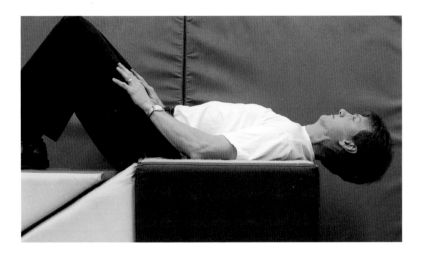

For flexion-based strengthening, lie on your back with the neck free.

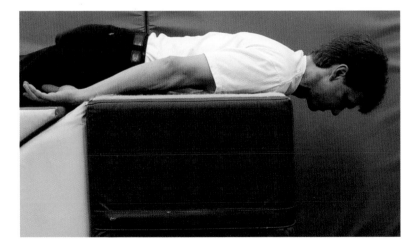

For extension-based strengthening, lie on your belly with the neck free.

PECTORALIS
STRETCHING EXERCISE

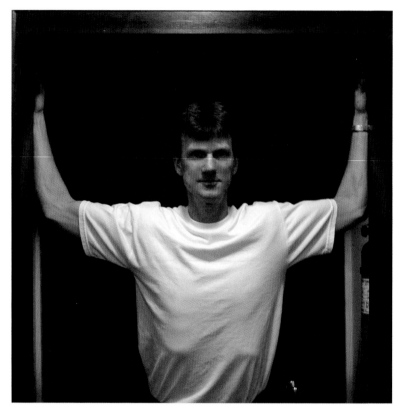

Use a door to stretch your pectoralis chest muscle. Scapula retraction is emphasized and strengthened and better posture is achieved.

POSTURAL EXERCISES USING LIGHT WEIGHTS

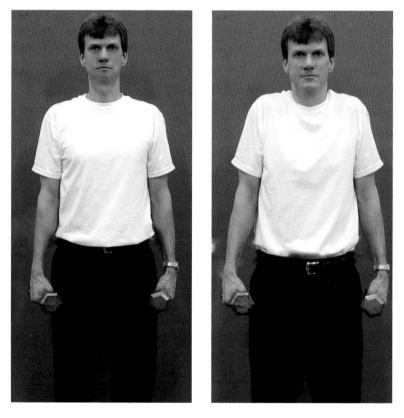

Exercises to accentuate good posture using light weights and multiple repetitions lead to further strengthening of the core neck muscles. In this exercise, the shrug is performed with light weights.

POSTURAL EXERCISES
USING THERAPEUTIC BANDS

E XERCISES TO ACCENTUATE GOOD POSTURE using therapeutic bands lead to strengthening of the core neck muscles.

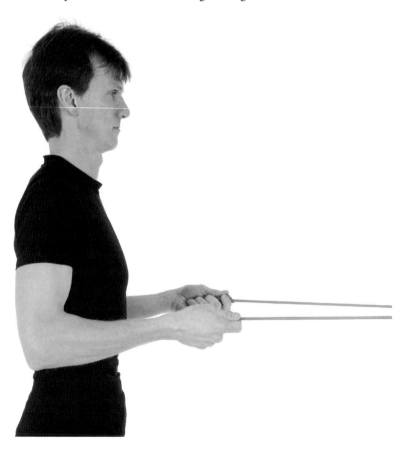

In this exercise, the core neck muscles that control scapula protraction and retraction are specifically strengthened.

RETURN TO CONTACT SPORTS/AGGRESSIVE PHYSICAL ACTIVITIES

O NE OF THE CRITICAL questions surrounding rehabilitation of the cervical spine in professional athletes is "when may I return to contact sports?" This is a similar question to a laborer in a high-demand position asking to return to the jack hammer, for example, after cervical spine surgery.

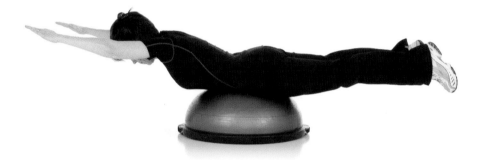

Typically the patient does not have a significant neurological deficit, and has been cleared for rehabilitation. Return to contact sports or aggressive physical activities usually occurs when they are able to demonstrate proficiency with resistance exercises on a ball. This decision is made jointly by the physical therapist and the surgeon.

BIBLIOGRAPHY

Murphy DR. *Sensorimotor training and cervical stabilization.* In: Murphy DR (ed.) Conservative Management of Cervical Spine Syndromes. New York: McGraw-Hill, 1999:607-640.

CHAPTER 12

Osteopathic Manipulative Medicine

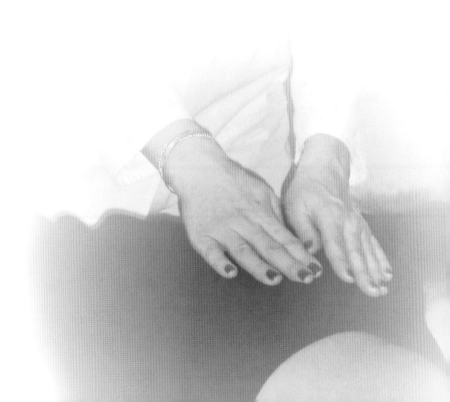

OSTEOPATHIC MANIPULATIVE MEDICINE

ANDREW TAYLOR STILL, M.D., D.O., was the founder of Osteopathy. Born in Virginia in 1828, his father was a doctor and a Methodist preacher. Initially, Dr. Still trained for 5 years to become an engineer, but subsequently attended the Kansas City School of Physicians and Surgeons around 1855. He became disillusioned with conventional medicine due to his medical experiences during the war, combined with the tragic loss of his three children that died during an epidemic of spinal meningitis.

Dr. Still developed osteopathic principles and techniques in his search for a better way to practice. The principles he founded were the interconnectedness of mind, body and spirit, the body's innate ability to heal itself, and the inter-relationship between the body's structure and function. Dr. Still defined osteopathy as, "that science which consists of such exact, exhaustive, and verifiable knowledge of the structure and function of the human mechanism, anatomical, physiological and psychological, including the chemistry and physics of its known elements, as has made discoverable certain organic laws and remedial resources, within the body itself, by which nature under the scientific treatment peculiar to osteopathic practice, apart from all ordinary methods of extraneous, artificial, or medicinal stimulation, and in harmonious accord with its own mechanical principles, molecular activities, and metabolic processes, may recover from displacements, disorganizations, derangements, and consequent disease, and regained its normal equilibrium of form and function in health and strength."

It is important to note that osteopathic manipulative treatment (OMT) is only one facet of osteopathic medicine. An osteopathic physician may use OMT alone or in combination with medications, surgery, rehabilitation, diet and exercise.

Autobiography of A.T. Still, A.T. Still, Kirksville, Missouri, 1908,

OSTEOPATHIC
MANIPULATIVE TREATMENTS

OSTEOPATHIC PHYSICIANS define soma or body as consisting of bones, joints, muscles, fascia, nerves, blood vessels and lymphatics. From time to time these systems become restricted leading to somatic dysfunction. Osteopathic manipulative treatments engage these restrictions directly by engaging the restrictive barrier or indirectly by moving away from the barrier. Some treatments are active when the patient assists or passive when the physician moves the body parts.

1	**Myofascial Release**
2	**Strain/Counterstrain**
3	**Facilitated Positional Release**
4	**Muscle Energy**
5	**Cranial Osteopathy**

MYOFASCIAL RELEASE

MYOFASCIAL RELEASE is a type of soft tissue treatment used to diminish pain and restricted motion of muscles and fascia. This is an indirect technique that describes the movement away from the restricted barrier to obtain relaxation of muscles, increase circulation, and promote lymphatic drainage.

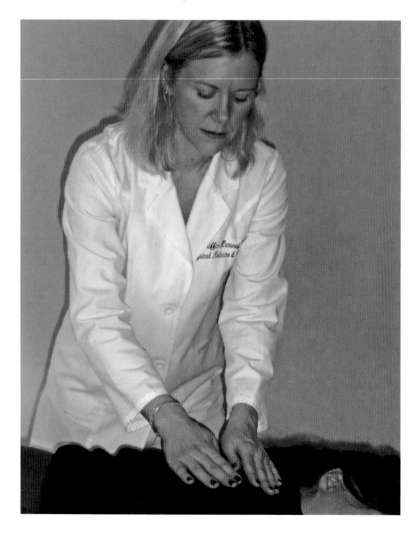

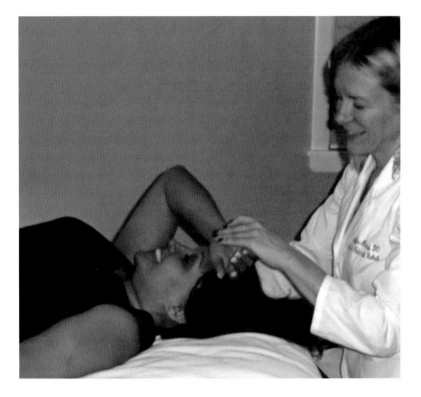

STRAIN/COUNTERSTRAIN

STRAIN-COUNTERSTRAIN was created by Dr. Lawrence Jones in the early 1960's. This technique is a positional release that reduces pain due to muscle and other soft tissue tightness. The somatic dysfunctional area is positioned at a point of balance away from the restricted barrier and in a shortened position for 90 seconds. This position of rest allows the pain cycle to break, resets muscle fibers and initiates the healing process.

FACILITATED POSITIONAL RELEASE

S TANLEY SCHIOWITZ, D.O., founded, developed and taught facilitated positional release (FPR) treatments to reduce soft tissue tension and release deep muscles involved in joint mobility. FPR is an indirect myofascial release technique in which the dysfunctional region is slowly moved into a neutral position in all planes and an activating force of torsion or compression is added.

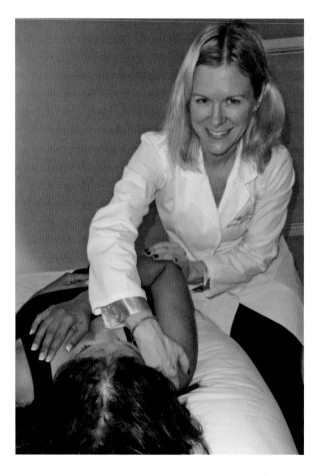

MUSCLE ENERGY

MUSCLE ENERGY directly addresses somatic dysfunctions by engaging the restricted barrier. The dysfunctional region or joint is taken into its barrier in all planes followed by the patient applying an equal and opposite force for 3-5 seconds. An increase in motion is noted and a new barrier is engaged and held. This is followed by the patient's brief counterforce once again. With this alternating treatment of contraction and relaxation, an improvement in range of motion is usually observed.

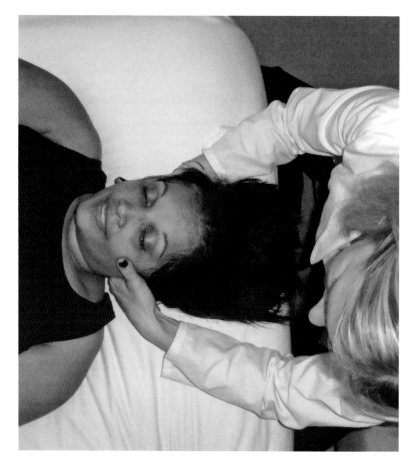

CRANIAL OSTEOPATHY

WILLIAM GARNER SUTHERLAND, D.O., is the founding father of Cranial Osteopathy who developed and taught this treatment in the early to mid-1900s. He emphasized during these years of practice that the Cranial Concept was an adjunct not a replacement to Dr. Andrew Still's science of osteopathy. Dr. Sutherland first perceived a very subtle, rhythmic movement present in the cranium and throughout the body. After years of studying, he named this phenomenon, "The Primary Respiratory Mechanism."

Osteopathic physicians trained in cranial treatments are able to palpate this cranial rhythmic, involuntary impulse that ebbs and flows independent of other body rhythms such as heart rate and breathing rate. A skilled osteopathic physician can directly connect with their hands to the patient's primary respiratory mechanism to elicit a therapeutic response.

Cranial osteopathic treatments include an intense feeling of deep relaxation, reset muscle fibers, break pain and stress cycles, and allow the body's innate ability to restore and heal itself.

CHAPTER 13

Yoga

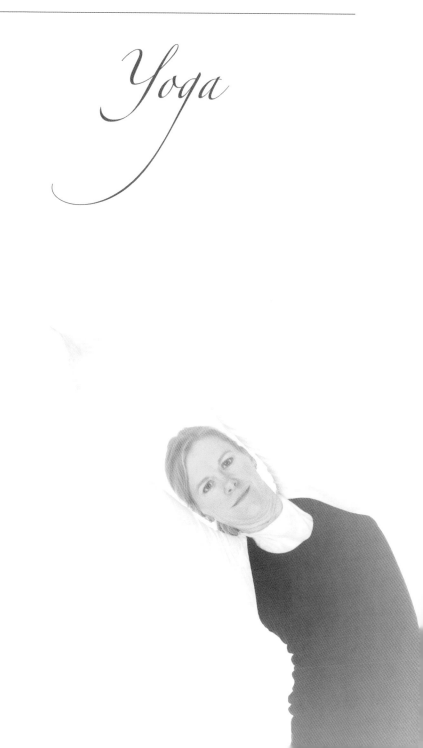

YOGA

YOGA IS THE SECRET WEAPON OF GREAT ATHLETES, EXTREME ATHLETES, GREAT ACTORS, MODELS AND HUMAN BEINGS SEARCHING FOR PHYSICAL AND SPIRITUAL INSPIRATION.

MENTALLY, YOGA ACKNOWLEDGES and services all of the body parts. The exercises lead to secretion of endorphins which support a deep sense of well-being. Deep breathing and respiration are integral aspects of yoga. Indeed with yoga you are taught to hyper-inflate your lungs bringing more oxygen to the human body. Your heart feels and performs better with yoga exercise.

Most yogic techniques emphasize range of motion of the facet joints. Most of the motion for the positions of yoga are facet joint based. The facet joints are then best serviced and perform optimally. Yoga leads to a limber and flexible spine which is, by itself, a definition of youthfulness. Spinal nerves benefit from the mobility of the exercises, the nerve mobility accompanying deep breathing, and the optimal status of the facet joints, which provides a roof for the nerve roots leaving the spine.

Body organs perform better with yoga. For example, with yogic movements and positions, gastrointestinal tract motility is improved. Predominantly, people engaging in the practice of yoga are very careful about their diet. They tend to prefer a plant-based green and leafy diet which in itself leads to better bowel movements and bowel health. Studies show better results in management of type 2 diabetes and menopausal symptoms with the use of yoga.

Extreme and endurance athletes rely on yoga postures for building strong muscles. Having a conversation with the rangers that patrol the New York harbor lead to the revelation of one of their great strength secrets. The rangers advised me that they perform 90 minutes of yoga per weekday in preparation for ice rescues, which requires strength, flexibility and balance.

Patients suffering with neck pain are best advised to start slowly with yoga. Deep breathing techniques and gentle range of motion activities under guidance of an instructor would be sufficient for starting. When symptoms abate, strengthening and postural yoga techniques may be undertaken with the clearance of your spinal physician.

Yoga poses with awareness of breath encourages highly-effective strength and flexibility training from poses held in stillness, and also in fluid sun salutation sequences. Expect to spend 6 months in training to develop a new body.

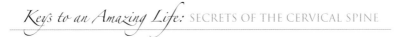

SEATED FLEXION
AND EXTENSION

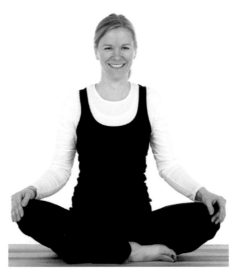

Sit with legs folded in front of you.

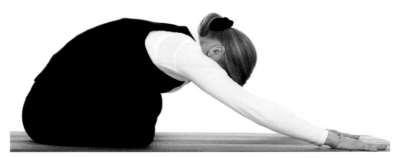

Reach forward with your arms,
feel each spinal facet joint release.

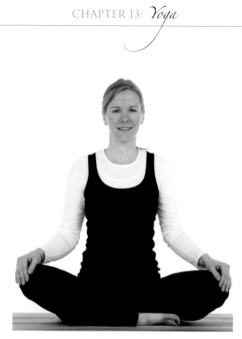

Sit with legs folded in front of you.

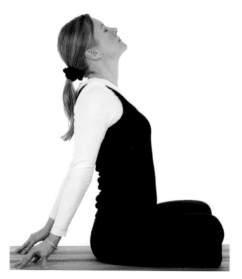

Reach backwards with your arms,
feel each spinal segment tighten a little bit.

SEATED RANGE OF MOTION

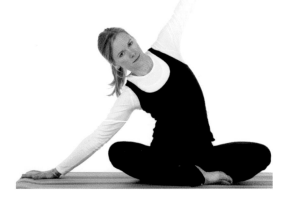

Plant the right hand on your mat, left arm is raised.
Feel the spinal facet joints open up on the left.

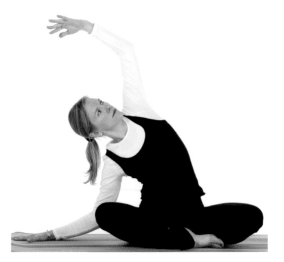

Slowly lean fully over to the right, feel each spinal
segment release on the left side of the body.

REPEAT ON THE LEFT SIDE

SEATED TWISTS

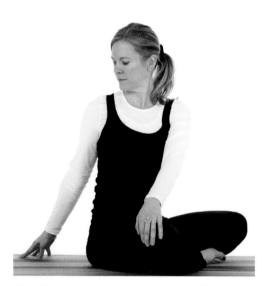

Seated rotation on the right rotates the facet joints
throughout the spine. You might hear a slight clicking sound.

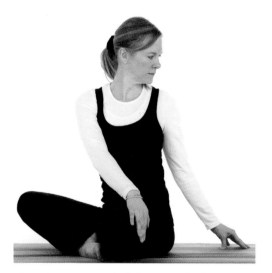

Seated rotation on the left rotates the facet joints
in the opposite direction. Rotate to a comfortable
position. You should not have pain.

SUN SALUTATION
(SURYA NAMASKARA)

A SUN SALUTATION IS A SERIES of hatha yoga movements and poses. The sequence of poses may be used as a form of exercise in which breathing techniques are essential. The incorporation of prayer and meditation may be used as a form of spiritual practice.

Sun salutations are usually performed in the morning to start your new day. This regime is usually performed in sets of 2, up to 8 at a time. While this series of movements salutes the sun, from the vantage point of the sun the human being is saluted. This ritual involves intention, respect of nature, deep breathing, spirituality, and whole body motion with attention to the core abdominal organs and muscles.

There are many variations of sun salutations with different movements for specific needs, enjoyment, and/or levels of difficulty. The reader will be presented in this chapter with a basic series of movements for bringing limberness, strength, and whole body movement with improved alignment and symmetry.

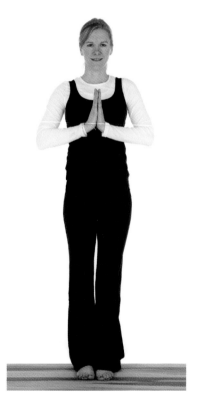

1. STANDING IN PRAYER POSE
Stand on mat with body erect and feet close together. Take a few breaths with hands in prayer position in front of chest.

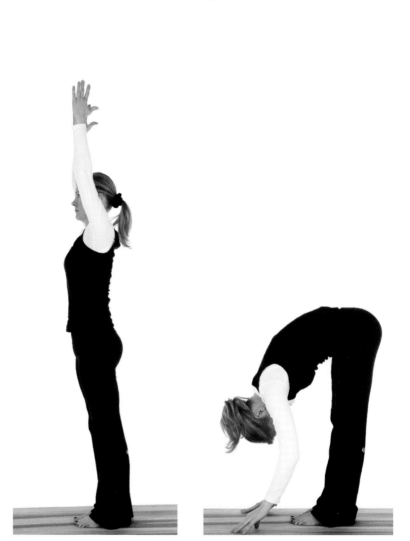

2. STANDING ARM REACH

As you inhale, raise your hands above head stretching abdomen, arms, and fingers. Tuck pelvis and keep arms in alignment with ears. One may arch backwards slightly to shine the heart center toward the sun.

3. STANDING FORWARD BEND

As you exhale, bend the upper body forward. Stretch the palms to touch your toes. May bend knees slightly if necessary.

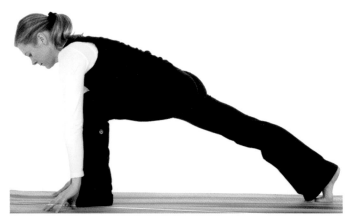

4. FORWARD LUNGE/LOW LUNGE

As you inhale, gently kick out the right leg while keeping the left knee bent with left foot between hands. The light touch of the fingertips to the ground with strong arms forces the core muscles to stabilize the body in this position.

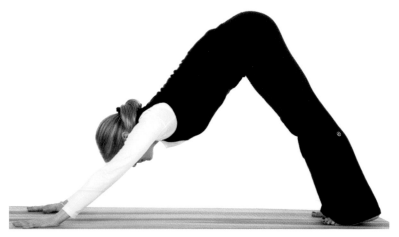

5. DOWNWARD DOG

As you exhale, form an upside down "V" with hips in the air and spine straight. Spread fingers and plant hands firmly on the ground. May peddle feet at first then work toward planting heels on the ground without changing foot placement.

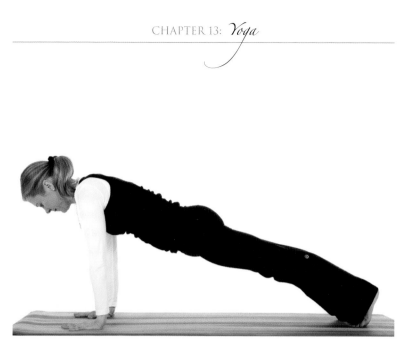

6. PLANK

Bring left leg to meet right leg in a push-up position. Keep neck in alignment with the spine and allow to gaze straight ahead.

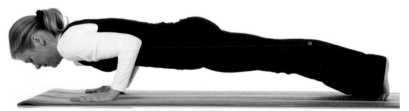

7. PLANK PUSH-UP

As you exhale, slowly lower the chest in a push-up position.

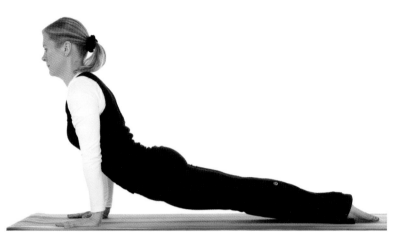

8. UPWARD DOG

As you inhale, scoop body forward with hands planted below shoulders. Tops of feet placed on mat. May lift hips and thighs off floor as seen in the picture.

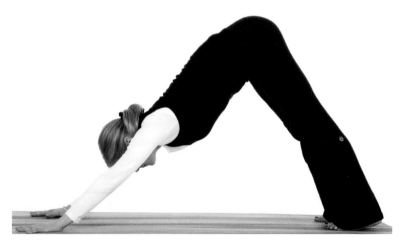

9. DOWNWARD DOG

As you exhale, form an upside down "V" with hips in the air and spine straight. Spread fingers and plant hands firmly on the ground. Same as in figure 5, may peddle feet at first then work toward planting heels on the ground without changing foot placement.

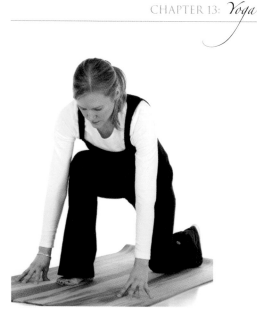

10. FORWARD LUNGE / LOW LUNGE

As you inhale, bring the right leg forward with right foot planted between the hands. The outstretched left leg may be bent slightly as shown in this picture or in a full leg extension with toes planted as in figure 4.

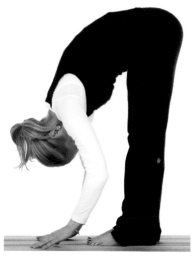

11. STANDING FORWARD BEND

As you exhale, bring left leg to meet right in a forward bend. Stretch the palms to touch your toes.

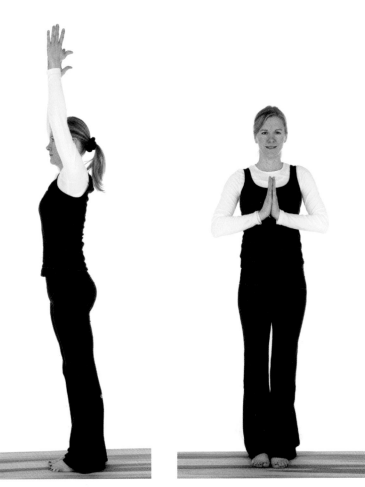

12. STANDING ARM REACH

As you inhale, raise hands above head stretching abdomen, arms and fingers. Tuck pelvis and keep arms in alignment with ears. One may arch backwards slightly.

13. STANDING IN PRAYER POSE

As you exhale, bring hands down into prayer position in front of chest. Maintain grounded foot position with good alignment.

Start the sequence again with Step 1. Except this time begin with left foot being kicked back in Step 4 and bring left foot forward in Step 10 in order to keep the body symmetrical and balanced as best as possible. Repeat the sun salutations 2–6 times as tolerated.

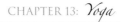
BIBLIOGRAPHY

Carter C, Stratton C, Mallory D. *Yoga to treat nonspecific low back pain.* AAOHN J. 2011 Aug; 59(8):355-61; quiz 362. doi: 10.3928/08910162-20110718-01. Epub 2011 Jul 25

Curtis K, Osadchuk A, Katz J. *An eight-week yoga intervention is associated with improvements in pain, psychological functioning and mindfulness, and changes in cortisol levels in women with fibromyalgia.* J Pain Res. 2011;4:189-201. Epub 2011 Jul 26.

Hegde SV, Adhikari P, Kotian S, Pinto VJ, D'Souza S, D'Souza V. *Effect of 3-Month Yoga on Oxidative Stress in Type 2 Diabetes With or Without Complications: A controlled clinical trial.* Diabetes Care. 2011 Oct;34(10):2208-10. Epub 2011 Aug 11.

Joshi S, Khandwe R, Bapat D, Deshmukh U. *Effect of yoga on menopausal symptoms.* Menopause Int. 2011 Sep;17(3):78-81.

Morone NE, Greco CM. *Mind-body interventions for chronic pain in older adults: a structured review.* Pain Med. 2007 May-Jun;8(4):359-75.

Parshad O, Richards A, Asnani M. *Impact of yoga on haemodynamic function in healthy medical students.* West Indian Med J. 2011 Mar;60(2):148-52.

Posadzki P, Ernst E. *Yoga for low back pain: a systematic review of randomized clinical trials.* Clin Rheumatol. 2011 Sep;30(9):1257-62. Epub 2011 May 18.

Sherman KJ, Cherkin DC, Erro J, Miglioretti DL, Deyo RA. *Comparing yoga, exercise, and a self-care book for chronic low back pain: a randomized, controlled trial.* Ann Intern Med. 2005 Dec 20; 143(12):849-56.

Sibbritt D, Adams J, van der Riet P. *The prevalence and characteristics of young and mid-age women who use yoga and meditation: results of a nationally representative survey of 19,209 Australian women.* Complement Ther Med. 2011 Apr;19(2):71-7. Epub 2011 Feb 8.

Yogitha B, Nagarathna R, John E, Nagendra H. *Complimentary effect of yogic sound resonance relaxation technique in patients with common neck pain.* Int J Yoga. 2010 Jan;3(1):18-25.

CHAPTER 14

Pain Management

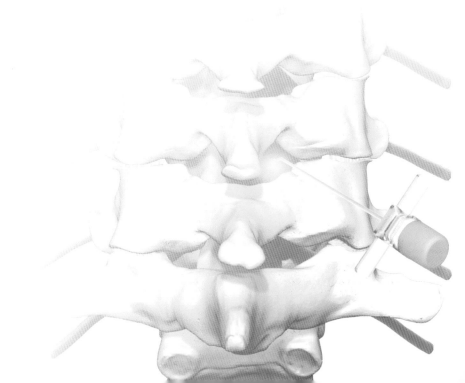

PAIN MANAGEMENT

PAIN MANAGEMENT specialists are doctors that are certified to relieve pain using injections and sometimes medications including narcotics. Pain management doctors typically do an extra year of training in the form of a pain fellowship. Anesthesiologists, Neurologists, Physical Medicine and Rehabilitation Specialists, or Psychiatrists typically choose to sub-specialize in the area of pain.

Working with your spinal physician, a pain management specialist might choose to try various injections to bring you relief. These injections are usually out-patient surgeries. While the injection is not as complicated as doing spinal surgery, it is still a procedure. Precautions as defined in the preoperative evaluation segment for surgery later in this book must be taken.

The pain specialist might offer you many types of interventions. The most common are:

1) Cervical Epidural Steroid Injection
2) Cervical Facet Block
3) Cervical Dorsal Rhizotomy = Radiofrequency Ablation

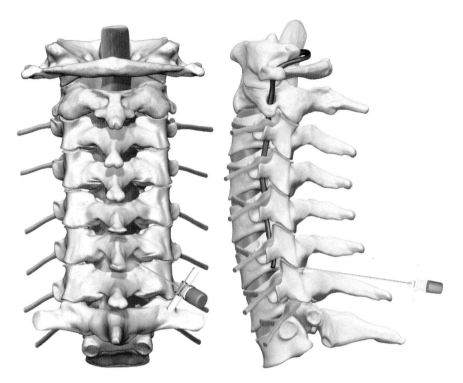

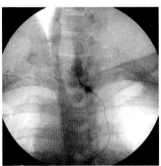

CERVICAL EPIDURAL STEROID INJECTIONS are injections of anesthetics such as lidocaine or marcaine combined with a steroid. The combination of medicines are placed in the epidural space. This epidural space is in between the ivory colored lamina (bony spinal canal) and the yellow colored dura (the soft tissue that contains the spinal cord and the spinal fluid called the cerebrospinal fluid). Decreasing the inflammation could be remarkably effective in diminishing pain and restoring function. Injections may last days to months. I find better results when the injections are combined with physical therapy. The patient needs to be carefully observed, postoperatively. Rarely, patients will suffer temporary complications such as loss of sensation, loss of motor power, or loss of blood pressure control.

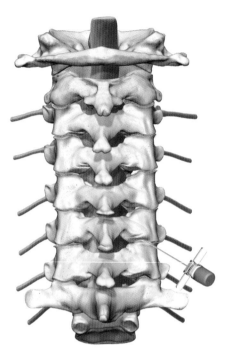
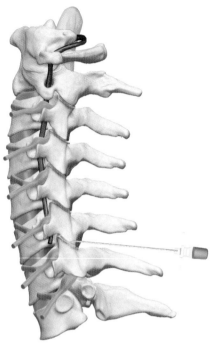

CERVICAL FACET JOINT INJECTIONS are injections of anesthetics such as lidocaine or marcaine combined with a steroid. The combination of medicines are placed into the facet joint. Facet joint pain manifests in the facet joints as neck pain and does not usually spread distally into the arms.

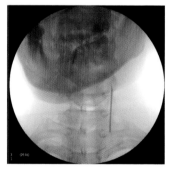

The facet joint is innervated by the medial branch of the dorsal ramus of the spinal nerve. The course of this nerve innervation is very consistent. Pain relief during the local anesthetic phase of this block is diagnostic of facet syndrome. The injections could be remarkably effective in diminishing pain and restoring function. The patient needs to be carefully observed, postoperatively. Rarely, patients suffer temporary complications such as loss of sensation, loss of motor power, or loss of blood pressure control, and are, therefore, observed after surgery.

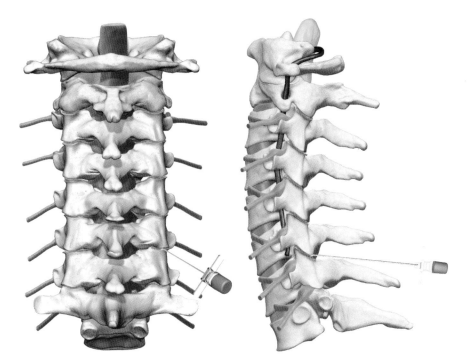

CERVICAL RADIOFREQUENCY DENERVATION aka DORSAL RHIZOTOMY: If the facet block brings temporary relief then the pain management specialist might offer a radiofrequency ablation procedure. Facet joint pain manifests in the facet joints as neck pain and does not spread distally into the arms. The facet joint is innervated by the medial branch of the dorsal ramus of the spinal nerve. Radiofrequency ablation is a treatment where the dorsal ramus of the spinal nerve that supplies the facet joint is ablated with heat used from a high frequency alternating current.

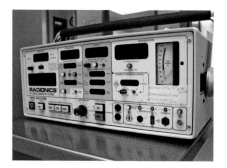

This stops the ability of the nerve to send a message to the brain that there is a deformed facet joint generating pain. This treatment might work for 12 to 18 months. That is enough time for this little nerve to regenerate. The patient needs to be carefully observed, postoperatively. Rarely, patients suffer temporary complications such as loss of sensation, loss of motor power, or loss of blood pressure control, and are, therefore, observed after surgery.

CHAPTER 15

Anterior Cervical Spine Surgery

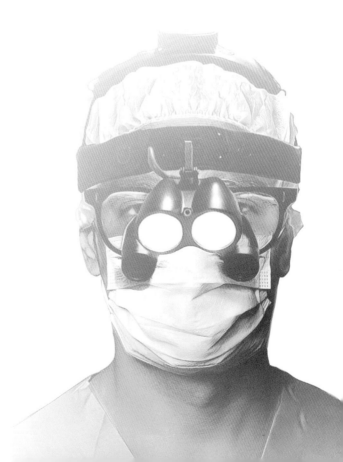

ANTERIOR CERVICAL SPINE SURGERY

ANTERIOR CERVICAL SPINE SURGERY describes operations that are undertaken from the front part of the neck. The decision to go anterior is driven by the nature of the problem, where the problem lies (anterior versus posterior), the level and extent of disease, and the surgeon's preference and comfort. The anterior approach is the work horse of neck procedures. It is most commonly used and it typically supplies a bloodless plane to work.

INDICATIONS FOR SURGERY

IMMEDIATE SURGERY	Severe neurological manifestations
	Progressive neurological deficits
ROUTINE SURGERY	Intractable pain
	Persistent neurologic deficit
	Severe postural shifting
	Failure of conservative treatment
	Recurrent irritation of the nerve

PREOPERATIVE EVALUATIONS

EVALUATION	EVALUATOR	CONSIDERATIONS
Radiographic Evaluation	Radiologist	X-rays, MRI's, Cat Scans, CT-Myelogram
Neurology Evaluation	Neurologist	Identify spinal and specific nerve problems. EMG
Physical Medicine & Rehabilitation Medicine	Physical Medicine & Rehabilitation Medicine	Functional considerations. Identify spinal and specific nerve problems. EMG
Basic Medical Evaluation	Family Practitioner Internist	Heart, Lungs, GI Tract, Whole Body
Vascular Evaluation	Vascular Surgeon	Arteries and Veins
Cardiac Evaluation	Cardiologist	Heart
Hematology Evaluation	Hematologist	Anemia, Consideration for blood production
Jehovah's Witnesses	Surgical Coordinator	Conscience categories including albumin and clotting factors. Use of erythropoietin. Cell Salvage – Jehovah's Witness protocol
Other Evaluations	As necessary	As necessary

MEDICATIONS: All patients who are taking aspirin or aspirin-containing compounds and/or non-steroidal anti-inflammatory medications, medications that promote blood thinning, and herbs should DISCONTINUE use for a period of TEN (10) days prior to the surgery date. **This has to be done in compliance with your medical doctor.** Any of the above medications have the potential of adversely affecting the surgical procedure, causing increased bleeding. NOTE: If, however, special circumstances require that the patient take these medications, it should be discussed with his/her medical doctor in advance.

A recent report stated that omega-3 and fish oil supplements taken up to 2 days before surgery do not cause increased bleeding during spinal decompression surgery.

SMOKING: All patients scheduled for a fusion should stop smoking as far in advance of the surgery as possible and continue to abstain during the post-operative period (until fusion heals 6–12 months). Studies show that smoking inhibits the formation of fusion bone.

REPORTED COMPLICATIONS

COMPLICATIONS Anterior Cervical Spine Surgery	ACDF Kostas et al. 1015 Patients	ACDF Cervical Spine Research Society 3428 Patients
Dysphagia	9.5%	
Postop hematoma = bleed	5.6%	
Cerebrospinal fluid leak	0.5%	
Esophageal Injury	0.3%	
Vertebral Artery Injury		
Spinal Cord Injury		0.2%
Vocal Cord Paralysis Laryngeal Nerve Palsy	3.1%	
Infection	0.1%	
Respiratory & Airway Complications		
Graft/Plate Construct Failures	0.1%	1 to 2%
Bone Graft		1.64%
Neurological worsening	0.2%	0.64%
Mortality = Death	0.1%	0.34% to 0.96%

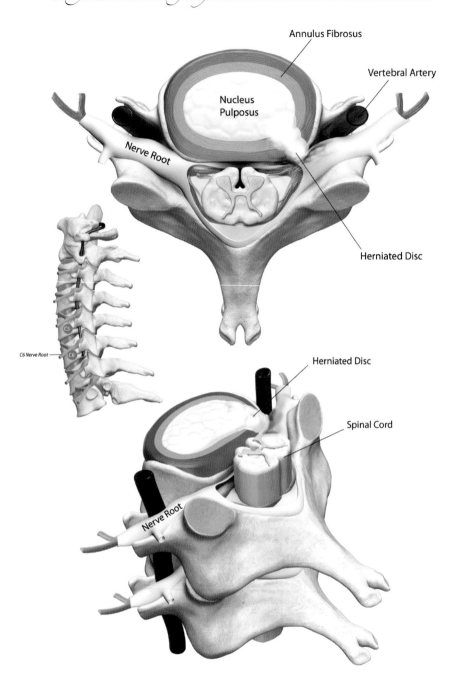

THIS IS AN EXAMPLE OF A C5-C6 HERNIATION
REQUIRING SURGERY

DECOMPRESSION

As surgeons, there are only a few options of procedures that we can offer to you. Decompression is the surgical strategy to debride or clean up an area. There are many varieties of decompressions offered, however.

In the case of this herniation, the disc must be removed. This figure shows the disc being removed with a pituitary rongeur.

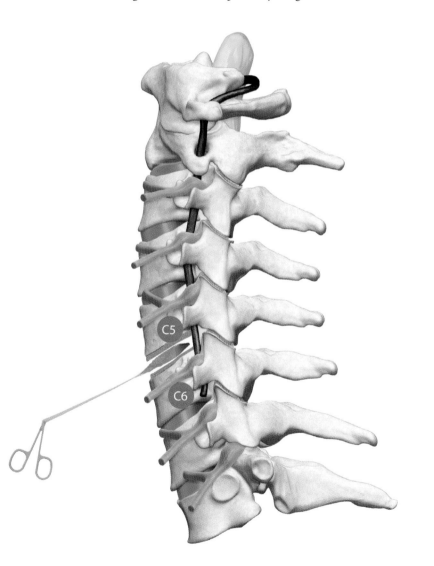

DECOMPRESSION

To aide the removal of the disc, the lower endplate of the C5 and the upper endplate of C6 are burred with a high speed drill. All arthritic fragments are also debrided.

From a geometric point of view, I remove a little bit more of the lower endplate of C5 and a little bit more of the upper endplate of C6 to allow for squaring of the vertebral bodies and a more stable placement of the bone graft.

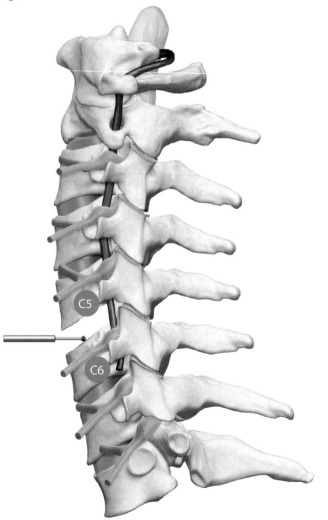

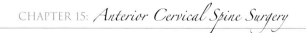

DECOMPRESSION

With the disc removed,
followed by the removal
of the spinal ligament, the
spinal cord becomes visible.

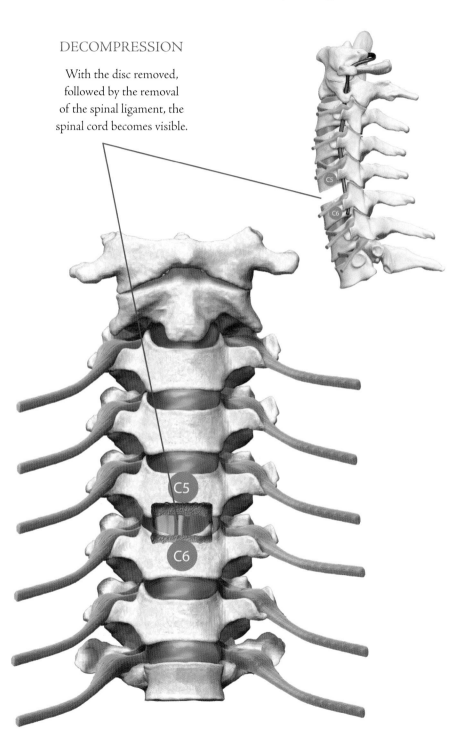

FUSION

Fusion, also known as arthrodesis, is the surgical technique to join two or more vertebrae using bone. Bone graft takes the form of:

+ Autograft (your own bone usually harvested from the pelvis)
+ Allograft (donor bone harvested from another human being, tested for diseases, processed and then available in specific sizes).

Smokers should not use donated bone since there is a significantly diminished chance of healing the bone graft.

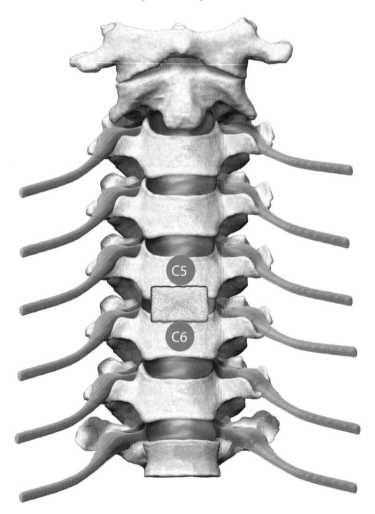

SPINAL INSTRUMENTATION

Spinal instrumentation refers to the use of metallic devices to hold two or more vertebrae in place. Provision of stiffness to the spinal segments allow the bone to fuse.

Spinal instrumentation allows the segment to be without motion. This promotes bone fusion.

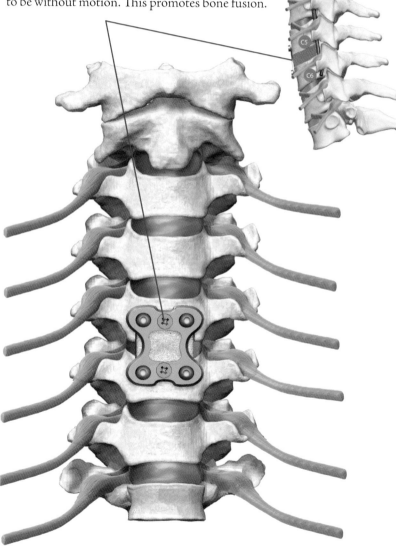

POSTOPERATIVE EVALUATIONS

MEDICATIONS: All patients who stopped taking aspirin or aspirin-containing compounds and/or non-steroidal anti-inflammatory medications, medications that promote blood thinning, and herbs may resume TEN (10) days after the surgery date. **This has to be done in compliance with your medical doctor and your surgeon.**

All fusion patients should know that anti-inflammatory drugs inhibit the healing of fusions and therefore anti-inflammatories should not be taken during the post-operative period (until fusion heals 6-12 months). It is important to use other medication to control pain other than the anti-inflammatories that are commonly prescribed for pain in the post-fusion cases.

The postoperative course is a very special time and presents unique opportunities. For the first time in a long time, the patient experiences pain relief from the structural removal of a blockage in the spine. Patients are usually pleased with the speed with which they could wean themselves off of narcotics. Besides having pain relief, patients find that for the first time in their life there is free time. Many patients walk 3 to 5 to 10 miles a day. Combined with a great diet, they lose excess weight and are feeling good about themselves.

In Hospital	Collar on at all times. Walk with assistance. Sit as tolerated with support. Avoid excessive spinal motion. Rolling (no twisting) encouraged.
1–2 Days	Barring any complications patient is discharged. Upon discharge the patient should be able to walk and climb stairs. Avoid bending, lifting, twisting or reaching.
1–4 Weeks	Walk as much as gently tolerated, and as many times in the day as tolerated. Avoid bending/lifting/twisting/reaching. Physical therapy in the form of massages and modalities may be administered in collar.
4–8 Weeks	Resume activities of daily living. The collar comes off at the surgeon's discretion – usually 4 to 8 weeks. When the collar is off, consider physical therapy, and may resume non-manual work. When the collar is off, labor intensive work may be started as tolerated, if approved by your surgeon.
1–3 Months	Return to work considered. Return to simple sports activities, especially in regards to walking, stationary biking and treadmill walking. Torsional activities such as tennis or golfing may take up to 9 months or longer, depending on progress.

SPECIFIC ACTIVITIES	DETAILS	BENCHMARK
Walking	Almost immediately after surgery First with an assistant/ Physical Therapist	1 day
Thinking Work	Discuss with surgeon	1 week
Stationary Biking	After collar is removed	6 weeks
Swimming	After collar is removed	6 weeks
Driving	After collar is removed Patient off of narcotics	6 weeks
Bending, Lifting, Twisting & Reaching in a controlled fashion	After collar is removed	6 weeks
Physical Sex	After collar is removed	6 weeks
Physical Therapy	After collar is removed	6 weeks
Physical Work	Discuss with surgeon, Physical Therapist input helpful	6 weeks – 3 months
Contact Sports	After collar is removed Start with progressive intensive physical therapy Clearance based on physical therapist & surgeon	3 months

Returning to work is a special decision to be made by the surgeon and the patient. Some executives are back to making decisions a few days after surgery. In other cases, it could be a few weeks. All patients are different and respond differently. Returning to thinking or physical work must be discussed and cleared with the surgeon.

Returning to contact sports is a decision made by the physical therapist and the surgeon. Typically, the surgeon approves physical therapy at 6 weeks. The physical therapist then clears the patient, progressively, using strategies such as cervical stabilization activities. When the athlete is able to perform resistance activities on an exercise ball, for example, then the physical therapist and the surgeon might clear the athlete to return to contact sports.

BIBLIOGRAPHY

Ang-Lee MK, Moss J, Yuan CS. *Herbal medicines and perioperative care.* JAMA. 2001 Jul 11; 286(2):208-16.

Fountas, Kostas N. MD, PhD; Kapsalaki, Eftychia Z. MD; Nikolakakos, Leonidas G. MD; Smisson, Hugh F. MD, FACS; Johnston, Kim W. MD, FACS; Grigorian, Arthur A. MD, PhD; Lee, Gregory P. PhD; Robinson, Joe S. Jr MD, FACS. *Anterior Cervical Discectomy and Fusion Associated Complications.* Spine: 1 October 2007 - Volume 32 - Issue 21 - pp 2310-2317

Graham, Jacob. *Complications of Cervical Spine Surgery: A Five-Year Report on a Survey of the Membership of the Cervical Spine Research Society by the Morbidity and Mortality Committee.* Spine: October 1989 - Volume 14 - Issue 10 - ppg 1046-1050

Kepler CK, Huang RC, Meredith D, Kim JH, Sharma AK. *Omega-3 and Fish Oil Supplements Do Not Cause Increased Bleeding During Spinal Decompression Surgery.* J Spinal Disord Tech. 2011 Mar 16. [Epub ahead of print]

CHAPTER 16

Posterior Cervical Spine Surgery

POSTERIOR CERVICAL
SPINE SURGERY

POSTERIOR CERVICAL SPINE SURGERY describes operations that are undertaken from the back part of the neck. The decision to go from behind is driven by the nature of the problem, where the problem lies (anterior versus posterior), level and extent of disease and surgeon's preference and comfort.

INDICATIONS FOR SURGERY

IMMEDIATE SURGERY	Severe neurological manifestations Progressive neurological deficits
ROUTINE SURGERY	Intractable pain Persistent neurologic deficit Severe postural shifting Failure of conservative treatment Recurrent irritation of the nerve

PREOPERATIVE EVALUATIONS

EVALUATION	EVALUATOR	CONSIDERATIONS
Radiographic Evaluation	Radiologist	X-rays, MRI's, Cat Scans, CT-Myelogram
Neurology Evaluation	Neurologist	Identify spinal and specific nerve problems. EMG
Physical Medicine & Rehabilitation Medicine	Physical Medicine & Rehabilitation Medicine	Functional considerations. Identify spinal and specific nerve problems. EMG
Basic Medical Evaluation	Family Practitioner Internist	Heart, Lungs, GI Tract, Whole Body
Vascular Evaluation	Vascular Surgeon	Arteries and Veins
Cardiac Evaluation	Cardiologist	Heart
Hematology Evaluation	Hematologist	Anemia, Consideration for blood production
Jehovah's Witnesses	Surgical Coordinator	Conscience categories including albumin and clotting factors. Use of erythropoietin. Cell Salvage – Jehovah's Witness protocol
Other Evaluations	As necessary	As necessary

MEDICATIONS: All patients that are taking aspirin or aspirin-containing compounds and/or non-steroidal anti-inflammatory medications, medications that promote blood thinning, and herbs should DISCONTINUE use for a period of TEN (10) days prior to the surgery date. **This has to be done in compliance with your medical doctor.** Any of the above medications have the potential of adversely affecting the surgical procedure, causing increased bleeding. NOTE: If, however, special circumstances require that the patient take these medications, it should be discussed with his/her medical doctor in advance.

A recent report stated that omega-3 and fish oil supplements taken up to 2 days before surgery do not cause increased bleeding during spinal decompression surgery.

SMOKING: All patients scheduled for a fusion should stop smoking as far in advance of the surgery as possible and continue to abstain during the post-operative period (until fusion heals 6-12 months). Studies show that smoking inhibits the formation of fusion bone.

REPORTED COMPLICATIONS

COMPLICATIONS Posterior Cervical Spine Surgery	Posterior Cervical Spine Research Society 3428 Patients
Postop hematoma = bleed	
Cerebrospinal fluid leak	
Spinal Cord Injury	1.5%
Infection	
Respiratory & Airway Complications	
Graft/Rod Construct Failures	1 to 2%
Bone Graft	0.39%
Neurological worsening	2.18%
Mortality = Death	0.34% to 0.96%

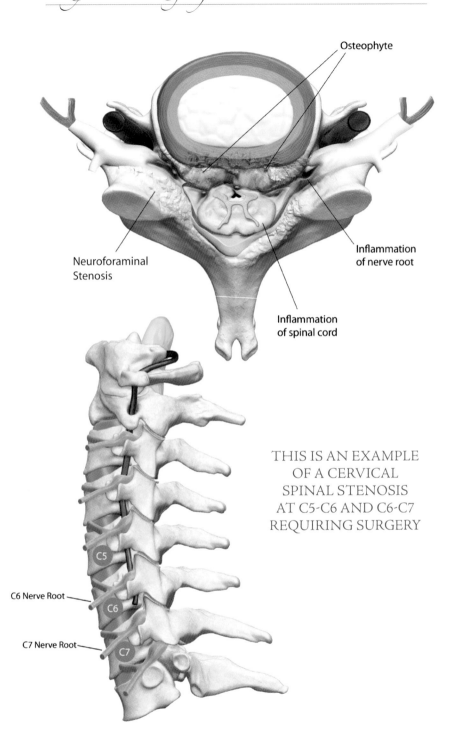

Osteophyte

Neuroforaminal
Stenosis

Inflammation
of nerve root

Inflammation
of spinal cord

THIS IS AN EXAMPLE
OF A CERVICAL
SPINAL STENOSIS
AT C5-C6 AND C6-C7
REQUIRING SURGERY

C5

C6 Nerve Root

C6

C7 Nerve Root

C7

DECOMPRESSION

In the posterior aspect of the neck we, as surgeons, might offer to debride or clean up a tight area.

Laminectomy is the procedure of removing the lamina and spinous processes. This procedure takes the pressure off the spinal canal.

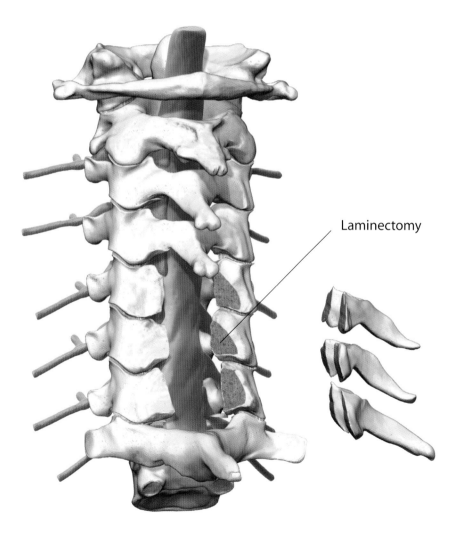

Laminectomy

DECOMPRESSION

Foraminotomy is the procedure of making more space in the neuroforamen. This procedure takes the pressure off specific nerve roots.

This figure shows the keyhole shaped opening made to decompress the nerve. Sometimes a herniated disc could be decompressed from underneath the nerve.

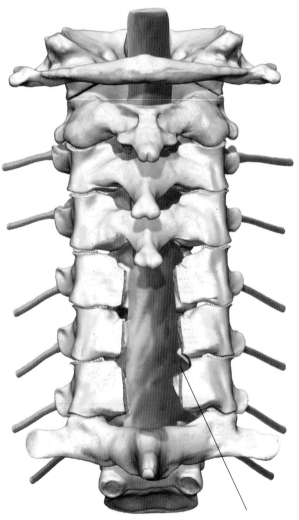

Neuroforaminotomy

FUSION = ARTHRODESISIS

Arthrodesis (arthro = joint, desis = to stop or stand) describes the stopping of motion at the facet joint.

Fusion is the laying down of bone graft on the surface of the previously operated bone. The bone consolidates into a solid fusion mass with time, permanently stopping motion.

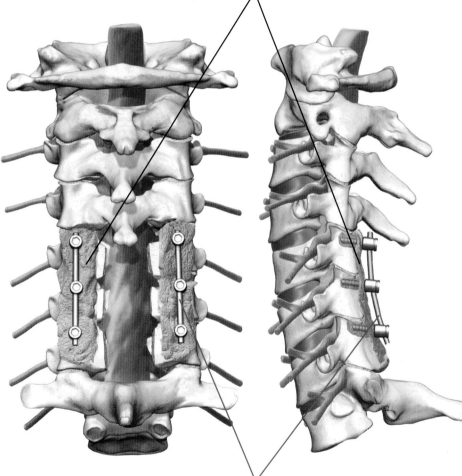

INSTRUMENTATION

Spinal instrumentation is used to immobilize spinal segments in order to allow spinal fusion to occur.

POSTOPERATIVE EVALUATIONS

MEDICATIONS: All patients who stopped taking aspirin or aspirin-containing compounds and/or non-steroidal anti-inflammatory medications, medications that promote blood thinning, and herbs may resume TEN (10) days after the surgery date. **This has to be done in compliance with your medical doctor and your surgeon.**

All fusion patients should know that anti-inflammatory drugs inhibit the healing of fusions and therefore anti-inflammatories should not be taken during the post-operative period (until fusion heals 6-12 months). It is important to use other medication to control pain other than the anti-inflammatories that are commonly prescribed for pain in the post-fusion cases.

The postoperative course is a very special time, and presents unique opportunities. For the first time in a long time, the patient experiences pain relief from the structural removal of a blockage in the spine. Patients are usually pleased with the speed with which they could wean themselves off of narcotics. Besides having pain relief, patients find that for the first time in their life there is free time. Many patients walk 3 to 5 to 10 miles a day. Combined with a great diet, they lose excess weight and are feeling good about themselves.

In Hospital	Collar on at all times. Walk with assistance. Sit as tolerated with support. Avoid excessive spinal motion. Rolling (no twisting) encouraged.
1–2 Days	Barring any complications patient is discharged. Upon discharge the patient should be able to walk and climb stairs. Avoid bending, lifting, twisting or reaching.
1–4 Weeks	Walk as much as gently tolerated, and as many times in the day as tolerated. Avoid bending/lifting/twisting/reaching. Physical therapy in the form of massages and modalities may be administered in collar.
4–8 Weeks	Resume activities of daily living. The collar comes off at the surgeon's discretion – usually 4 to 8 weeks. When the collar is off, consider physical therapy, and may resume non-manual work. When the collar is off, labor intensive work may be started as tolerated, if approved by your surgeon.
1–3 Months	Return to work considered. Return to simple sports activities, especially in regards to walking, stationary biking and treadmill walking. Torsional activities such as tennis or golfing may take up to 9 months or longer, depending on progress.

SPECIFIC ACTIVITIES	DETAILS	BENCHMARK
Walking	Almost immediately after surgery First with an assistant/ Physical Therapist	1 day
Thinking Work	Discuss with surgeon	1 week
Stationary Biking	After collar is removed	6 weeks
Swimming	After collar is removed	6 weeks
Driving	After collar is removed Patient off of narcotics	6 weeks
Bending, Lifting, Twisting & Reaching in a controlled fashion	After collar is removed	6 weeks
Physical Sex	After collar is removed	6 weeks
Physical Therapy	After collar is removed	6 weeks
Physical Work	Discuss with surgeon, Physical Therapist input helpful	6 weeks – 3 months
Contact Sports	After collar is removed Start with progressive intensive physical therapy Clearance based on physical therapist & surgeon	3 months or more

Returning to work is a special decision to be made by the surgeon and the patient. All patients are different and respond differently. Returning to thinking or physical work must be discussed and cleared with the surgeon.

Returning to contact sports is a decision made jointly by the physical therapist and the surgeon. Typically, the surgeon approves physical therapy at 6 weeks. The physical therapist then clears the patient, progressively, using strategies such as cervical stabilization activities. When the athlete is able to perform resistance activities on an exercise ball, for example, then the physical therapist and the surgeon might clear the athlete to return to contact sports.

BIBLIOGRAPHY

Ang-Lee MK, Moss J, Yuan CS. *Herbal medicines and perioperative care.* JAMA. 2001 Jul 11; 286(2):208-16.

Graham, Jacob. *Complications of Cervical Spine Surgery: A Five-Year Report on a Survey of the Membership of the Cervical Spine Research Society by the Morbidity and Mortality Committee.* Spine: October 1989 - Volume 14 - Issue 10 - ppg 1046-1050

Kepler CK, Huang RC, Meredith D, Kim JH, Sharma AK. *Omega-3 and Fish Oil Supplements Do Not Cause Increased Bleeding During Spinal Decompression Surgery.* J Spinal Disord Tech. 2011 Mar 16. [Epub ahead of print]

INDEX